ENGINEERING IN THE HEART AND BLOOD VESSELS

WILEY INTERSCIENCE SERIES
ON BIOMEDICAL ENGINEERING

Advisory Editor: JOHN H. MILSUM, McGill University

Geddes and Baker
Principles of Applied Biomedical Instrumentation

Myers and Parsonnet
Engineering in the Heart and Blood Vessels

ENGINEERING IN THE HEART AND BLOOD VESSELS

GEORGE H. MYERS

Head, Biomedical Engineering Laboratory,
Riverside Research Institute
Adjunct Professor of Electrical Engineering,
New York University

VICTOR PARSONNET

Director of Surgery and Chief of Vascular Research,
Newark Beth Israel Medical Center
Clinical Associate Professor of Surgery,
New Jersey College of Medicine and Dentistry

WILEY-INTERSCIENCE

a Division of John Wiley & Sons
New York · London · Sydney · Toronto

Library of Congress Catalogue Card Number: 70-77837

SBN 471 62722 4

Printed in the United States of America

To Our Wives

Foreword

"To love,
is not to gaze steadfast
at one another:
it is to look together
in the same direction."

St. Exupery, "Terre des Hommes"

Biomedical engineering is but one of many new interdisciplinary endeavors of great importance to us—important because their study and exploitation provide almost our only hope of finding acceptable compromise solutions to our increasingly complex sociotechnological problems. Of course, the different disciplines of science have always cross-fertilized one another to some extent, but until recently science's explosive growth has tended necessarily to fragment our knowledge into somewhat isolated compartments. This specialization, however, has been so successful in the generation of new knowledge and technological capacity that now one of our desperate needs is to synthesize this knowledge into socially useful groupings; for example, groupings to tackle the problems of the pollution of resources, and of political, ecological, urban and transportation, and health systems.

The synthesizing process seldom continues for long without causing some practical difficulties for the people involved. Each discipline has inevitably acquired its own "language" and set of basic assumptions and constraints and, of course, some "mystique" as well. Further, there may be considerable resistance against the retrenchment of individual disciplines necessary for new ones to be synthesized from some of their parts. Indeed sound arguments may also be advanced to show that experts from several disciplines are required to work in concert in complex problems, such as those already mentioned, and thus to achieve a crude form of "intelligence amplification." It would seem that both methods will be necessary; that is, interdisciplinary collaboration can coexist fruitfully with new synthetic disciplines.

A basic attribute of either method is expressed in the words of St. Exupery, quoted above: "to look together in the same direction," even if from different points of view. The present series in BioMedical Engineering is therefore addressed to this need.

Books in the BioMedical Engineering series will be published to educate persons of one discipline in what they need to know of others and to catalyse a synthesis in the core subject generally known as biomedical engineering. Thus one set of titles will aim at introducing the "classically trained" biologist and medical scientist to the quantitatively based analytical theories and techniques of the engineer and physical scientist. This set covers instrumentation, mathematical modeling, signal and system analysis communication and control theory, and computer and simulation techniques.

A second set is intended for engineers and physical scientists and covers basic material on biological and medical systems with a presentation as quantitative and compact as possible. The omissions and simplifications necessitated by this approach should be justified by the increased ease of transferring the information and more subtly by the increased pressure it can bring to bear on the search for unifying quantitative principles.

Some subjects of biomedical engineering interest will be treated in texts of considerable depth, whereas fast-changing subjects will be treated in monographs. Typical areas include biomaterials, prosthetic systems, ecological modeling, systems identification, and computer-aided diagnosis.

Medicine is being forced more and more into the public spotlight in direct relation to its increasing power to affect the quality and quantity of human life. Biomedical engineering is contributing significantly to these developments and must also be responsibly concerned with the inevitable social questions of "what, to whom, and when and where." This series therefore will also focus on the social correlates of biomedical engineering, for only in this way, I believe, can the theoretical benefits of technological advance be assured of transformation into real, practical benefits for humans in their complex imperfect societies.

John H. Milsum
Préville, Quebec
November, 1968

Preface

This book is devoted to the technological, device-oriented aspects of artificial internal organs in the human cardiovascular system. The cardiovascular system has become an area in which in recent years many engineering techniques, both theoretical and technological, have been applied. In the theoretical area methods of mathematical analysis, which were formerly reserved for determining the transfer functions of guided-missile systems, have now been applied to determining the method by which the body regulates blood pressure. Instrumentation developed for the space program has been widely used in these efforts in order to make the necessary measurements, and the electronic computer has become a fixture in the medical laboratory, as well as a tool for medical practice. As a result of the recent emphasis on theory medical education is beginning to change in a number of institutions, with much more emphasis on physics and mathematics. It is not unusual to see physicians taking courses in differential equations in some medical schools.

However, it seems fair to say that much of the interest in the theoretical side of the human body has been sparked by the need for new knowledge for the design and development of new devices. The cardiac pacemaker is perhaps the most successful application of electronics to the design of a prosthetic, and its use has created an entire new industry. However, optimum application of the cardiac pacemaker in all of its specialized forms required a much more thorough understanding of the mechanisms of rate control and the electrophysiology of the heart, and so this device has been indirectly responsible for much theoretical research. Similarly, the problems arising with the current program to develop an artificial heart have led to extensive theory on how the human heart itself operates and also to much study on the effects of implants in the human body.

The principal devices discussed are the pacemakers, the artificial heart, heart valves, and vascular prostheses. These devices are covered from three aspects. First, there is a description of the pertinent physiology of the "natural" human organ, written so that those untrained in biology can understand the material. Second, there is a summary of the basic operating principles of the most important of the devices of the class (including many in the research stage). Third, there is a review of the materials used in the implanted devices, in which particular attention is given to their properties in a biological environment. Numerous tables and experimental data are included in this category.

No attempt has been made for several reasons to give a complete analysis of the numerous devices described. A complete book would be necessary to do each justice, and in many cases this book has already been written. Also, much of the material would be out of date in a very short time. Rather the approach here has been to indicate the general working principles of each of the devices, along with the relative problems and advantages, and to show the areas in which future improvement may be expected. Thus the researcher or clinician in the field may learn the general methods of operation and the theoretical principles of new devices. He will also have data on the physiology and materials involved.

George H. Myers
Victor Parsonnet

New York, New York
Newark, New Jersey
May 1969

Acknowledgment

The person who probably had the most to do with the creation of this book is Mr. Evan Herbert of "Science and Technology Magazine." He suggested the topic for the magazine article which was the predecessor to this book and greatly encouraged us to expand the material into its present form. His encouragement persuaded us that a book of this kind would be useful and helpful.

In the course of writing the manuscript numerous others have been of great assistance. Foremost among them are our colleagues at the Newark Beth Israel Medical Center: Dr. E. L. Rothfeld, Dr. I. R. Zucker, Dr. L. Gilbert, and Mr. Thomas Coullahan, who prepared many of the illustrations. Mrs. Charlene Kessler, who typed the manuscript, deserves special thanks. Miss Beatrice Shube, our editor at John Wiley and Sons, provided much help and encouragement when it was needed, and Dr. Howard Gadboys of Mount Sinai Medical Center, who unfortunately died during the preparation of this manuscript, was most helpful to us.

G. H. M.
V. P.

Contents

ENGINEERING IN THE HEART
AND BLOOD VESSELS

CHAPTER ONE

Artificial Internal Organs

Faulty organs can be replaced or transplanted from another person (or an animal) or by an artificial organ, a prosthesis. Whereas it would appear simpler to use organs from other individuals (homotransplantation) rather than artificial devices, the homotransplantation method has the problem (aside from that of availability of "spare parts") that the natural defense mechanisms of all living organisms, the immune reaction, reject foreign matter, and in particular foreign proteins. Reducing the effectiveness of the immune reaction by drugs or radiation increases the susceptibility of the subject to infection, and thus has its own special set of hazards. Therefore the best type of kidney transplantation, for example, that can be done with high assurance of success (about 90%) is from identical twin to identical twin. Transplants from sibling to sibling and parent to child are less successful, and transplants between nonrelated donors are poorer still (about 25% success after one year). For these reasons much recent emphasis has been placed on the creation of artificial organs. It is possible to use for these devices materials that are accepted by the body, so the immune reaction does not cause any difficulties. However, artificial organs are not just like the "real thing," and therefore compromises are implicit in their use.

The basic medical engineering problem is to design a prosthesis that will be accepted by the body, has low power input, is small, and still has an acceptable working lifetime; for example, the present artificial kidney, to which a patient must be connected from time to time, is larger in size than a human torso. Artificial hearts, although often not much larger than a natural heart, require so much power to operate them that at the moment there does not seem to be any way of providing this energy internally with a predictable lifetime that would match the patient's life expectancy. Some research approaches to this problem will be described in detail later in this book.

The body interior is a hostile environment for materials, and for working electrical and mechanical parts. Body temperature is the only factor that is relatively constant. The liquid environment in which an artificial organ op-

1

erates is highly corrosive and is also an excellent conductor of electricity. Furthermore, the continuous motion of many parts of the body (e.g., the beating of the heart when it is connected to pacemaker wires for 24 hours a day) causes mechanical fatigue.

After complete implantation an artificial device is remote from instrumentation and control, even though it may be only a few millimeters beneath the surface of a subject's skin. Furthermore, the environment itself cannot be controlled. Initial design and experimental verification therefore must surmount this crucial barrier of unpredictability.

Prosthetic devices can, like circuit elements, be roughly classified as *passive* or *active*. Most of the passive organs, such as artificial bones or blood vessels, are structural elements and support devices. On the other hand, active devices supply energy to parts of the body, and may therefore be regarded as being involved in the body's metabolic processes. The outstanding example of an active device is the cardiac pacemaker, with which much of this book is concerned. The artificial heart is another example of an active prosthesis, since it too supplies power in order to pump blood. In this classification artificial heart valves would be passive, since they do not require energy input.

The energy for all active prostheses has until now come from implanted batteries, by electromagnetic induction or radio-frequency energy transmission from outside the body, or from wires or tubes conducted through the skin. The body obviously generates sufficient power to operate the natural organs, and indeed the power output of most artificial devices is quite small. Thus, if electronic or mechanical devices could be made efficient enough, it would be possible to operate them with no external sources. Means for accomplishing this are currently a field of active research, and are described in detail.

A problem shared by both active and passive prostheses is body acceptance. Blood clots can develop in artificial blood vessels, deposits can form around electrodes, and scar tissue developing about implants is an almost universal process. From experience it has been found that some types of metals—such as 300-series stainless steels, tantalum, and noble metals—have good acceptance characteristics. Certain plastics are also fairly inert in the body and are widely used. Silicone rubber has such wide application that some forms of it are now classed as drugs and require approval of the Food and Drug Administration for their use. Teflon and Dacron are also quite inert and are used chiefly as blood-vessel substitutes.

Surprisingly, the roughness of the plastics used in artificial blood vessels is of considerable importance [1]. Early prostheses of this type were built with smooth interiors with the goal of preventing clots from adhering to the sides of the vessels. However, it turned out that smooth interior surfaces actually aggravated the clotting problem. An autogenous lining (one produced by the body) formed on the inner surface, and tended to peel off and plug the vessel. A similar phenomenon occurred with artificial heart valves, where a similar lining came loose and floated freely in the blood stream. In contrast, when the vessel is constructed of fabric the new lining adheres to it, and its interior becomes like that of a natural vessel. The rough, somewhat porous surface permits the lining to "stick" long enough for the fibrous tissue to grow into it, thereby incorporating the foreign material into the body [2]. A continuing problem with such artificial arteries is that the new lining decreases the diameter available for blood flow. If it is sufficiently small, the vessel may be closed up altogether. This has limited the use of textile grafts to vessels whose diameter exceeds several millimeters. Such artificial vessels have also not been successful in venous replacements. Evidently the low velocity of blood flow in veins causes sufficient clotting so that the flow is reduced completely.

The reaction just described illustrates that, although blood appears to be a simple fluid, it is actually quite complex, composed of many small, living cells. The crushing action of some early and even recent artificial hearts, heart-lung machines, and synthetic heart valves often badly damaged the blood cells [3]. Although it is now known how to minimize damage of this sort, it is still a considerable problem in the design of the artificial heart, which must be designed so that no metal comes in contact with the blood cells to minimize shearing forces on the cells. These constraints rule out, for example, the common piston pump.

Figure 1.1 indicates the status of the development of artificial internal organs as of this writing (1968) [4]. Some of the passive prostheses, especially those in the cosmetic category, are very old: artificial eyes and limbs have been known since antiquity. The conduits, such as blood vessels, are relatively new in their successful application, since they required both new materials and new surgical techniques. Research in these areas is principally one of finding new and improved materials. One important development in this area is the possibility of using *natural* materials to construct artificial blood vessels. For some time blood vessels have been transplanted from one part of the body to another in an attempt to overcome the immune reaction, but such a technique is limited by the fact that it is necessary to find either a replacement vessel that is not needed or to replace the replacement. It now appears that it is possible to insert tubes of solid plastic into the body in such a manner that scar tissue grows around them and forms a tube of natural material [5]. (This encapsulation has been referred to above.) The plastic tube can then be withdrawn, leaving an artificial blood vessel of nat-

® NEW
PEOPLE PARTS

Development stage	Regulators	Active Pumps	Conduits	Misc.	Filters	Conduits	Passive Supports	Fluids	Cosmetic
Now used internally in humans, self-contained power source	Heart valve, Cardiac pacemakers, Carotid (blood pressure) asynchronous stimulator, Phrenic stimulator			Hearing aid		Blood vessels, Trachea	Bones, Mesh for hernia, Tendons, Injected silastic Armatures, Brain membranes	Plasma substitute	Eyes, Teeth, Ear cartilage, Artificial breasts and testes
Now used experimentally in humans or animals	Carotid synchronous pacemaker, Bladder pacemaker, Self-energized cardiac pacemaker				Lung	Research on new materials	Research on new materials		
Used internally in humans but requires external power		Heart, Ventricle		Larynx	Kidney, Lung				
Connected to living system but used externally because of size and power requirements	Respiratory center	Heart-lung machine, Iron lung							
Proposed			Nerves, Peristaltic conduits	Kidney, Brain				Blood substitute	

← Development flow

Figure 1.1 Chart showing the present status of implanted artificial internal organs.

4

ural tissue. The technique is still experimental and has certain obvious draw-backs (e.g., it is necessary to wait until the plastic tube has become encased in the fibrous tissue), but it holds great promise. In effect, it is a technique by which the surgeon "grows" a special transplant inside the patient.

Although the passive prostheses are of great importance, the active prostheses are considerably more complex but hold the hope of being able to cure a wider range of diseases. Probably only one of these devices, the hearing aid, is truly widespread in its use. The hearing aid and others, such as the artificial kidney, the iron lung (actually an artificial diaphragm), and the heart-lung machine obviously are not truly internal organs but just replace the functions of internal organs by external means. The artificial heart cannot be said to be truly internal at this time, although much effort is being expended to make it so.

However, numerous stimulators are now achieving considerable importance. The most successful of these, the cardiac pacemaker, has now been implanted in an estimated 30,000 people in the United States and in many more abroad. The success of the cardiac pacemaker has led to the development of other types of stimulators—all of which are truly internal in that they are completely implanted within the body, and all are active.

A general characteristic of all pacemakers and other stimulators is that their power output is uniformly small, on the order of microwatts. Thus they act as biological "triggers." Some act to amplify and conduct a stimulus created in the body to a particular organ; others generate some of the information required to produce the correct pulses themselves. These extremes are exemplified by two types of cardiac pacemakers, the so-called synchronous and asynchronous pacers. The synchronous pacer detects the natural rhythmic electrical signal from the atria of the heart, which in heart block is not transmitted to the ventricles, and then applies a properly timed stimulus to the ventricles. The asynchronous pacemaker generates its own rate internally (the rate is usually preset by the manufacturer), irrespective of the natural rate-adjusting mechanism of the body.

The cardiac pacemaker is presently the most important of the various types of internal stimulators, both medically and commercially, and is given the greatest amount of attention in this book. It will serve as a model, both electronically and physiologically, for many other types of devices.

An example of such a related device is the carotid-sinus stimulator, which has often been inaccurately dubbed a baropacer. One of the more important ways in which blood pressure is regulated is by way of the carotid-sinus reflex arc. Pressure-sensitive receptors in the carotid sinus, located on the carotid artery in the neck, detect the blood pressure and transmit the information to the brain by way of the carotid-sinus nerve. The cardiac center in the medulla then interprets this information and sends out signals on efferent nerves to regulate the blood pressure either by changing the heartbeat (in rate or stroke volume) or by changing the diameters of the resistive blood vessels. It has been found that, by coupling electrical impulses onto either the nerve or the carotid sinus, blood pressure can be reduced; appropriate stimulators to do this already have been implanted in humans. Although this application is apparently completely different from that of the cardiac pacemaker (indeed, the device is not a pacemaker at all, since no speed is being regulated), it turns out that many of the basic problems that must be overcome are similar to those of the cardiac pacer. The carotid-sinus stimulator must solve the difficulties imposed by long-term implantation and by long-term electrical stimulation of a part of the body. The power output of the carotid-sinus pacer is of the same order of magnitude as that of the cardiac pacer (although the actual pulse rates, widths, and amplitudes are different) and therefore has similar power-conservation difficulties. The techniques in designing the electronics and in packaging them, as well as the problems involved with the leads that actually conduct the electrical stimulus to either the nerve or the heart, are almost identical.

The bladder stimulator is a voluntary efferent neuron, intended for use in paraplegic patients who cannot urinate because the nerves controlling the sphincter muscles in the bladder have been severed. The stimulator applies an electrical stimulus to the bladder or its nerves, on command from the outside, causing the sphincters to relax and the bladder to contract and force out the urine. The engineering problems involved here are not so severe as with the two types of pacemaker just described, because continuous operation is not required, which eases the power requirements. Body acceptance and encapsulation problems are the same, however.

Although the bladder stimulator corresponds to a voluntary neuron, note that the impulse for it to react does not come from the brain directly but from some other route, such as the patient's turning on a switch as a result of a signal from his brain. In the normal human urination is both voluntary and involuntary—except in infants, where it is entirely under reflex control; voluntary control is acquired through training. Similarly electronic stimulators may be used to regain control over other paralyzed muscles, such as those in the arm or the leg. A muscle or motor unit may be paralyzed if its neural connection to the brain in interrupted. Since the muscle and its terminal nerve fibers have not actually been damaged in such a case, the muscle maintains its contractability. However, after a period of disuse it will atrophy. For many years practitioners of physical medicine have been using electrical stimulation to prevent and delay atrophy; however, these measures, although they preserved the muscle, actually did nothing to restore its functions, because contact with the voluntary controlling nerve centers had been lost. Electrical stimulators to activate the nerve have been developed to perform this function.

A somewhat oversimplified description of how these devices work illustrates their activity and indicates possible avenues for future work. Suppose a man wishes to perform a complex motion, such as moving an object from one point to another. After he has decided to perform the action, a cerebral function, the command is passed to another cerebral center, which in turn directs various subcenters. The subcenters send appropriate impulses along the nerves to the appropriate muscles. In this example sensing organs in the tendons, muscles, joints, and the eye observe the movement and serve as measuring devices in the feedback loop. Therefore, when the effecting (efferent) nerve paths are damaged, the extremity becomes paralyzed. It is possible, however, that some other muscles, used for completely different purposes, still remain normally innervated (under normal control), and that these muscles are not used in everyday activities. Such a muscle might be, for example, an adductor muscle of the shoulder, which normally brings the arm inward. The functions of this muscle might not be affected by a spinal injury, and it does not play a vital part in everyday living. If, by means of learning, the cerebral pathway could be transferred from the normal one to the one controlling the still normal muscle, and if then an external bypass could be constructed so that, say, adducting the arm caused the leg to move, then the patient could regain control over his paralyzed muscle. The possibility of sensing control signals from the peripheral nerve path or brain centers has been considered but up to now has not proven feasible because of technical difficulties. Approaches that have met with success have been to detect the contractions of the muscle, either by external devices such as strain-gauges or potentiometers, or by use of the action potentials of the auxiliary muscles as control signals that regulate the stimulation of the desired muscle. The analogy to both the synchronous cardiac pacemaker and the bladder stimulator is obvious.

Restoration of breathing in paralyzed patients by means of the familiar iron lung (an externally applied artificial organ) is well known. The same function can be achieved by a device known as an electrophrenic stimulator, which can be used when the phrenic nerve is intact. Control of rate and depth of breathing is located in the respiratory center in the brain. Automatic involuntary respiratory movements are caused by the rhythmic discharge of nervous impulses from this center, which pass down the spinal cord and through the phrenic nerve to the diaphragm and through other nerves to auxiliary muscles of respiration. Proper electrical stimulation of the phrenic nerve causes respiratory movements, even in cases of paralysis (especially paralytic poliomyelitis), and stimulators have been constructed to perform this function [6]. The impulses have been led through the skin either by radio-frequency transmission or by wires (wires would probably not be satisfactory for long-term stimulation). Whereas some of these stimulators have had a fixed respiratory rate, others have had a manually adjustable control or servomechanisms with feedback loops activated by sensors that detect the oxygen and carbon dioxide content of the expired air.

All of the preceding examples of stimulators control what may be loosely called mechanical physiological functions. In general the stimulation either regulates or causes some motion, rate, or pressure. Many of the biochemical functions of the body are under nervous control, and therefore we would expect that electrical stimulation would be able to affect the chemical as well as the mechanical behavior of the body. As a matter of fact, it has been shown that the amounts of blood glucose and liver glycogen in rabbits are changed by electrical stimulation of the hypothalamus [7]. In the experiment reported, stimulation of the ventromedial hypothalamic nucleus (one of the nuclei in the sympathetic area of the hypothalamus) caused an increase in blood glucose followed by a pronounced decrease in liver glycogen.

The same investigators electrically stimulated the splanchnic nerve, the peripheral sympathetic nerve innervating the liver. They found that the activities of two enzymes (glycogen phosphorylase and glucose-6-phosphatase) were greatly increased within 30 seconds of the start of stimulation. It is probable that this changed enzyme activity was responsible for the changes observed when the hypothalamus was stimulated. The stimulation approximately tripled phosphorylase activity for the period in which stimulation was maintained. The activity of liver glucose-6-phosphatase was also increased about 40 percent.

Although the liver stimulator is more of a curiosity than a useful device, it illustrates a trend that may be observed in recent years; many therapeutic functions formerly considered to be in the field of drugs are now being treated by electronics. Before the advent of the cardiac pacemaker heart block was invariably treated with drugs, but in the last few years the treatment of choice has become the electronic pacemaker. Drug therapy is still the treatment used for hypertension, but now, for cases that are not amenable to this, the carotid-sinus pacemaker can be used. Medication for indigestion is commonplace; however, it has been suggested that certain types of intestinal activity can be aided by electrical stimulation, although it seems unlikely that electronic devices will ever replace any of the various pills and medications for an upset stomach. Many glands are under nervous control; it is conceivable that electrical stimulation could effect cures in cases where drugs cannot.

A truly encyclopedic volume would be required to discuss all of these devices in any sort of detail, but they all have one thing in common—they must supply electrical pulses at a certain rate, and with certain characteristics, to nerve or muscle fibers. The power requirements are all of the same order of magnitude; and they all have the same environment in the body, with the same attendant problems that are, incidentally, shared by passive artificial organs as well. The approach here is to treat the physiology of cardiac and carotid-sinus pacemakers in detail. The cardiac pacemaker is included because it is the most successful completely implantable artificial organ and has undergone the most sophisticated development. Also, since its proper function usually is a matter of life or death to the patient, proper understanding of all aspects of its application is important. The carotid-sinus stimulator is included because its application introduces a wide variety of problems that are encountered by other devices and because it is the subject of much research at the moment. Since the cardiac pacemaker is an example of muscle stimulation, and the carotid-sinus stimulator is an example of stimulation of a nerve, these two cases are actually amenable to considerable generalization.

Following this the technology of pacemakers is discussed both from a medical and an engineering viewpoint. The medical aspects include the different forms of pacing, such as synchronous versus asynchronous, myocardial versus endocardial electrodes, pacemaker placement, and side effects and complications of pacing. The electronics necessary to perform these functions is then discussed, followed by an analysis of the materials involved in encapsulation and the power problems involved in pacemaker life. The "gray area" between the medical and engineering problems is the interface between the electronics and the body: the point at which the stimulating electrodes contact the body. Many of the problems experienced with pacemakers seem to arise in the region; for example, it has been mentioned that the provision of power is a problem with pacemakers, because long battery life is desired. Recent work has shown that only a small fraction of the power supplied by a pacemaker to the heart is effective in stimulation. The rest is dissipated in a small region about the point where the electrode contacts the heart. Furthermore, this wasted power increases with time. Various electrochemical reactions occurring in this area are also responsible for decreased electrode life and other deleterious effects such as tissue necrosis. An attempt is made to give as complete a picture as possible of what is known about these phenomena and of what remains to be done.

The pacemaker at the moment is the most successful of the active internal organs. However, research in artificial hearts continues, and it seems likely that a working device will be available in the near future. Thus a large part of the remainder of the book is devoted to their description. One form of the artificial heart is actually a reality: the heart-lung machine used in open-heart operations. Although this device is not implantable (and therefore somewhat out of the scope of this book), it is covered in detail because it has acted as a model for much investigation into implantable hearts.

Materials used in implantable devices present a continuing problem. Much of the state of the art of biomedical materials is reviewed, especially where these properties affect the devices described. A discussion of materials naturally includes some of the passive implants (since these must be fabricated directly from suitable materials), and so the usefulness of various materials of these passive implants are discussed.

REFERENCES

[1]   Davila, J. C., "The Development of Artificial Heart Valves," *Plastics in Surgical Implants,* ASTM (American Society for Testing Materials), Spec. Pub. STP 386, 1964.

[2]   Edwards, W. S., *Plastic Arterial Grafts,* Thomas, Springfield, Ill., 1957.

[3]   National Academy of Sciences, *Mechanical Devices to Assist the Failing Heart,* NAS Pub. 1283, 1966.

[4]   Myers, G. H., and V. Parsonnet, "Engineering Inside the Body," *Int. Sci. and Technol.,* February 1965.

[5]   Parsonnet, V., and M. Khatami, "A New Animal Preparation for Measurement of Aortic Pressure and Flow," *J. Newark Beth Israel Hospital,* 18:222 (1967).

[6]   Sarnoff, S. J., E. Hardenbergh, and J. C. Whittenbager, "Electrophrenic Respiration," *Amer. J.* 155:1 (1948).

[7]   Shimazu, R., and A. Fukuda, "Increased Activities of Glycogenolytic Enzymes in Liver after Splanchnic-Nerve Stimulation," *Science,* 150:1607 (1965).

CHAPTER TWO

Physiology of Cardiac Rate Control

1. REGULATION OF THE HEARTBEAT

There are clearly two aspects of the regulation of heartbeat. The first is concerned with generating a signal to the heart to control its beat; the second is concerned with how the heart itself reacts to this signal. We consider first those external cardiac factors that regulate the heart rate.

The rate and force of the heartbeat are controlled by nerve impulses. The nerve impulses, which we shall consider first, are transmitted over the afferent and efferent fibers of the cardiac nerves, operating through the cardiac center located in the medulla oblongata. Although the heartbeat is basically an automatic action originating within the heart itself, nervous impulses acting reflexly can change the heart rate in response to body conditions.

Afferent fibers have two roles: they carry sensory impulses from the heart to the central nervous system, and they carry impulses from pressure sensitive receptor cells lying at the base of the aorta and in the carotid sinus, known as pressure receptors or baroreceptors. The sensory impulses from the heart have clinical significance, because pain impulses conducted by them can indicate inadequate blood supply to the heart. The baroreceptors play a key role in the maintenance of heart rate. They are called depressor fibers because, as blood pressure rises, they act reflexly to lower the blood pressure. There are also receptors in the large veins and the right atrium. Distension of these sensors by increased venous return causes impulses that reflexly increase the heart rate, and therefore these fibers are called pressor fibers. Both pressor and depressor fibers pass along the cranial nerves to the reflex centers of the medulla.

The baroreceptors, which are described in more detail in the next chapter, produce electrical impulses whose rate is proportional to both the absolute value of blood pressure and the rate of change of blood pressure. Each individual receptor produces its own train of impulses, and each receptor has different factors of proportionality relating the impulse rate to pressure and

11

rate of change of pressure. Since there are a large number of receptors at a particular location, examination of the output of a particular receptor site shows electrical impulses with irregular spacing. The intervals between the impulses become smaller on the average (on an oscilloscope they become denser) as the pressure increases.

The heart receives nerve impulses through two sets of afferent fibers, both of which belong to the autonomic nervous system. These are the right and left vagus nerves (of the parasympathetic division) and the accelerator nerves (of the sympathetic division). Both the vagus and the accelerator nerves exhibit tone; that is, they exert a continuous effect on the heart. Nerve impulses from centers in the brain are continuously being discharged over the vagus, exerting their restraining influence to decrease heart rate. Simultaneously, and also continuously, the heart is receiving impulses over the accelerator nerves, which tend to increase its rate [1].

Nervous control of the heart is effected primarily by the cardiac center, which is located in the medulla in the floor of the fourth ventricle. From a portion of this area, the cardio-inhibitory center, impulses are discharged through the vagus nerves to the heart; from another portion, the cardio-accelerator center, impulses travel down the spinal cord to the upper thoracic region, then by way of spinal nerves and sympathetic ganglia through accelerator nerves to the heart.

Chemical substances in the blood also play a role in the control of heartbeat. Of importance is a proper balance of various ion concentrations in the blood and tissue fluids. If there is calcium excess, the heart stops in systole (calcium rigor—intense spasm). In the case of sodium excess the heart becomes progressively weaker and finally stops in diastole (a relaxed state). Potassium excess produces effects that are similar to those caused by sodium excess.

In addition to these substances, carbon dioxide and oxygen tension in the blood have important effects on heart rate. A slight excess of carbon dioxide tension stimulates the vasoconstrictor center of the brain, bringing about constriction of the peripheral blood vessels. Blood pressure rises, and the heart is reflexly slowed as a result of the stimulation of the baroreceptors. A great excess of carbon dioxide decreases the tone of the cardio-inhibitory center and decreases impulse conduction in the atrioventricular bundle, with resulting slowing of the heart. Overventilation, which reduces carbon dioxide tension in the blood, causes an increase in heart rate. Excessive increase of hydrogen ions, such as occurs in acidosis, causes a block in the electrical impulse pathways in the heart.

Low oxygen tension, like low carbon dioxide tension, increases the heart rate; however, if oxygen levels become excessive, irregularities in heart action occur. The rate becomes slower, and the heart fails. Interference with the oxygen supply to the heart muscle itself, as occurs in coronary artery obstruction, damages the heart.

Cardiac action is also affected by circulating chemicals (humoral agents) such as hormones. Epinephrine increases both the rate and force of ventricular contractions when applied to isolated hearts. When it is injected into the body, it raises blood pressure, which reflexly slows the heart. Thyroxin (thyroid hormone) also increases the rate of the heart.

Many drugs, especially alkaloids, affect heart action. Some produce their effects principally through their action on acetylcholine, which is produced at the vagus endings. Since this book is concerned principally with electrical phenomena in the heart, we shall not pursue the interesting field of chemical control, other than to mention it here.

Controls of the heart may be considered to be either *homeostatic,* or natural regulatory controls; or *disturbance* controls, which are involved in adapting the body to new circumstances. In general the phenomena discussed here have been homeostatic. Under a fixed set of circumstances the body's regulatory mechanism maintains oxygen pressure, carbon dioxide pressure, arterial-blood pressure, heart rate, and blood flow constant. Outside inputs, however, can alter the level at which these parameters are maintained; for example, exercise requires altering heart rate and blood flow in an attempt to maintain the oxygen in the tissues constant. Various diseased states also result in altered control levels.

2. THE HEARTBEAT

We have just briefly indicated how the rate of the heart and its contractions are controlled by the body as a whole. A major point of interest, however, is how these control functions are acted on within the heart.

The impulse that initiates the heartbeat starts in the sinoatrial (S-A) node, the natural pacemaker of the heart, which is less a point than a region, as may be seen in Figure 2.1. The S-A node is itself controlled by the vagus and accelerator nerves, which have just been discussed. Studies have shown that as the heart rate drops, the site of the electrical activity shifts to an area closer to the ventricles [2] (Figure 2.2).

From the S-A node an electrical excitation wave spreads through the muscle of the atria to the atrioventricular (A-V) node, which lies at the junction of the atrium and the ventricles. The excitation wave causes the atria to contract. At the same time the impulse is conducted through the atrioventricular node to the bundle of His and its branches to the ventricles. The

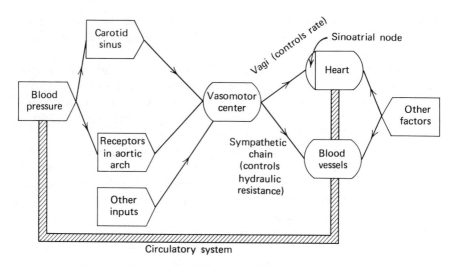

Figure 2.1   Block diagram illustrating pathways of cardiac control.

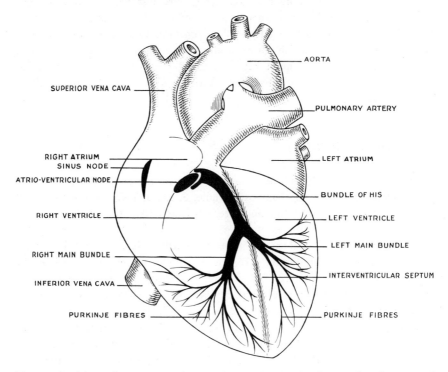

Figure 2.2   Schematic representation of human heart showing major features of conduction system.

bundle of His is a conducting tract that originates in the A-V node; its fibers pass into the ventricles and then excite virtually all cells of the ventricles. As a result, after the electrical impulse passes along this bundle to the muscle cells, both ventricles contract almost simultaneously. By contrast, in the atria the electrical wave passes progressively from one muscle cell to the next at a finite, relatively slow rate. As a result a gradual, coordinated contraction wave passes over the atria.

Complete interruption of the passage of the electrical wave through either the A-V node, the bundle of His, or its branches is called complete heart block. This produces a loss of the normally coordinated heartbeat. The atria continue to contract at their normal rate, but the impulses are not transmitted to the ventricles. Ventricular cells, however, are similar to the pacemaker cells of the S-A node in that they have an intrinsic electrical activity, but at a much slower rate (20 to 40 beats per minute). The ventricles then may continue to beat at this lower intrinsic rate, which is usually insufficient to prevent the serious consequences of an inadequate cardiac output. The artificial pacemaker is used to provide a more rapid rate.

3. EXCITATION AND CONDUCTION

The overall mechanism of the heartbeat and its control have been described from a phenomenological viewpoint, intended to give the reader a reasonable perspective of the overall physiological process. One important area that has direct importance for pacemakers and pacemaker research is the mechanism of electrical conduction in the heart cells, and the mechanism of their excitation. This is rightfully an entire field in itself, and several books have been written exclusively on this topic. It is pertinent, however, to give some idea of the mechanisms involved in these cell phenomena [2, 3, 4].

The primary event in the conduction of an impulse along an excitable fiber is the development of depolarization at the excited point of the cell membrane. Normally there is a positive charge outside and a negative inside the membrane. This depolarization excites the adjoining area of the membrane and thus continues down the length and breadth of the fiber. Depolarization is a change in potential between the outer membrane of the cell and its inside. The excited area is not only depolarized but its polarity is actually reversed.

Two phenomena are actually present: a conduction of an electrical impulse along a fiber, and a change in potential between the core and the exterior of a conducting cell, which is known as the action potential. The conduction

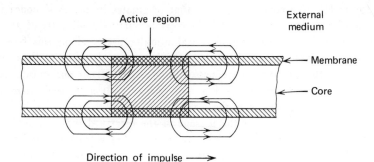

Figure 2.3   Relationship of local action potentials and propagation of a wave along a cell.

of an impulse along the cell is characterized by varying action potentials at different points. During the passage of an impulse, action currents flow in small, longitudinal loops, as shown in Figure 2.3. The net longitudinal current that flows through a cross section including both the inside and the outside of the cell is zero, but the current densities are not necessarily the same inside and outside. The axial current inside is concentrated in the core

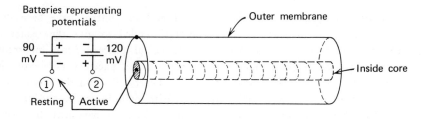

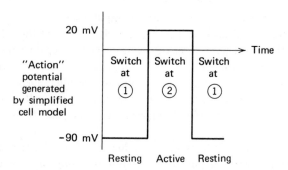

Figure 2.4   Equivalent circuit giving static representation of action potentials.

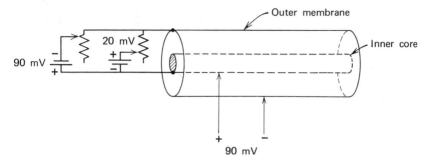

Figure 2.5 Equivalent circuit showing transmembrane resting potentials.

of the cell, whereas the currents outside are distributed in the extracellular fluid. The simplified model of the theory that we shall now present has been described in detail by Hoffman and Cranefield [3].

When an excitable cardiac fiber is at rest, its interior is about 90 mV negative with respect to the exterior. If the fiber is conducting an impulse, the inside of the fiber becomes about 20 mV positive with respect to the outside as the impulse passes. These phenomena may be represented by the "equivalent circuit" of Figure 2.4, in which a switch changes from one position to another as an impulse passes by. The so-called action potential indicated by this model would consist of a resting potential of 90 mV (inside negative) and an instantaneous reversal to 20 mV (inside positive) as the impulse passes, simulated by throwing the switch. Since the transition between these two states, however, is not actually instantaneous, some mechanism is needed for simulating the smooth transition that actually occurs. This can be done by using two variable resistances, as shown in Figure 2.5. The circuit of Figure 2.5 is more than just an interesting representation that happens to give the same potentials as the cells: it has an actual basis in fact. The source of the potential difference is the different concentration of sodium and potassium ions. If solutions containing unequal concentrations of K^+ are separated by a membrane selectively permeable to K^+, the potential across the membrane is given by

$$E_K = \left(\frac{RT}{F}\right) \ln \frac{K^+_i}{K^+_o}$$

or, at 37°C,

$$E_K = 61.5 \log_{10} \frac{K^+_i}{K^+_o} \text{ mV},$$

in which E_K is the potential difference caused by the differences in concentrations of K^+ inside and outside the membrane, represented by K_i^+ and K_o^+. The symbols R, T, and F represent the gas constant, absolute temperature, and the Faraday constant, respectively.

It is possible to obtain quite accurate measurements of the potassium concentration in some excitable tissues. Measurements in cat heart muscle lead to a value of $E_K = 92.6$ mV.

The distribution of Na^+ is opposite to that of K^+. There is more K^+ inside the cell than outside, whereas there is more Na^+ outside than inside. To be exact, the ratio of potassium inside to outside is 31, whereas the equivalent ratio for sodium outside to inside is 24. Using the formula just presented leads to a potential due to sodium of 84 mV, inside positive.

The question naturally arises as to how the cell maintains the differences in concentration of potassium and sodium, since we would expect the various potentials and concentration gradients to be such as to bring about equilibrium. As a matter of fact, the motion of sodium through the membrane goes against both concentration and electrical potential gradients. This is evidently due to an active, metabolic process, which has been given the name of the "sodium pump" [5]. The other ionic movements are conceivably passive.

Thus the values of the battery voltages in the equivalent circuit have been determined. In order to obtain a relation for the resistances let us consider one of the branches in the model of Figure 2.5, say the potassium branch, by itself, and examine the current through a short circuit across the cell wall. This will give, from Ohm's law,

$$E_K = I_K R,$$

where I_K is a current flow in which charge is carried by the movement of K^+ ions. If the source of the voltage is the unequal distribution of these ions and the corresponding current is carried by the movement of the ions, then the resistance term must correspond to the resistance to the flow of the ions through the membrane, and we may write

$$E_K = I_K R_K.$$

The resistance to a flow of a specific substance through a membrane is the reciprocal of the permeability, P_K, so $R_K = 1/P_K$. A similar procedure may be carried out for the sodium branch.

Although sodium and potassium are the major contributors to the transmembrane potentials, to be really accurate it is necessary to add an extra voltage source and resistance for other ion species and to add a capacitor to allow for membrane capacity. This model is shown in Figure 2.6, which con-

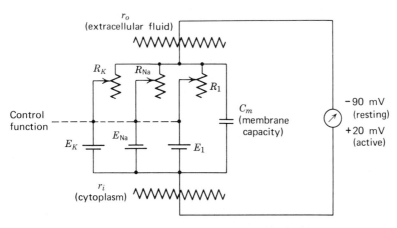

Figure 2.6 Equivalent circuit of cell showing factors necessary to explain activity and recovery.

tains all properties necessary to describe voltage changes associated with activity and recovery, except for the times involved.

It is only necessary now to consider the conduction properties from cell to cell to arrive at a picture of the whole heart surface. Both the extracellular fluid and the cytoplasm conduct electric current because of the presence of inorganic ions and also to some extent because of the presence of larger organic ions. The goal will be to derive an equivalent "transmission line" circuit of the body of excitable cells, as contrasted to deriving equivalent sources, which was the subject just considered.

The fact that a voltage difference of about 90 mV exists across the membrane of excitable cells indicates that the membrane has a resistance to current flow, which represents the permeability of the cell to charged ions. The

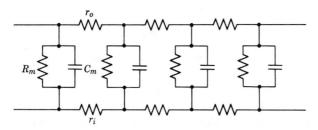

Figure 2.7 Equivalent circuit of a cell, using lumped approximation to distributed parameters actually found. Batteries representing various potentials have been omitted for clarity.

fact that capacitance also exists can be shown by suddenly applying a small current across the membrane of an excitable cell. It is found that the transmembrane potential does not change suddenly but reaches a new value rather slowly. At the polarizing electrode the voltage has an exponential waveform. The presence of both resistance and capacitance give a membrane what is called its core-conductor properties.

An excitable cell is more or less cylindrical and long with respect to its diameter. The cytoplasm and the extracellular fluid (which surrounds the cell) both conduct current. The presence of both resistance and capacitance means that the cell may be represented by the equivalent circuit of Figure 2.7, which may be recognized as the equivalent circuit of a transmission line without inductance. The transverse resistance of the membrane is higher than the longitudinal resistance of the extracellular fluid or cytoplasm, which means that the flow of current resulting from the application of a voltage at one point spreads along the length of the fiber, a phenomenon referred to as electrotonic spread.

The two cable properties of chief interest are the time constant and the "length" constant, which determines the rapidity of exponential drop along the cell, according to the relationship

$$P = P_0 \, e^{-x/\lambda},$$

where $x =$ the distance from the applied voltage,
$P =$ the change in voltage at x,
$P_0 =$ the applied change in voltage,
$e =$ the base of natural logarithms $= 2.71828 \ldots$,
$\lambda =$ the length constant.

Since only final steady-state values are considered in this expression, the membrane capacity does not affect the value of the measured potentials. The space constant for the Purkinje fibers, for example, is about 2 mm.

The membrane time constant τ_m is defined by

$$\tau_m = R_m \, C_m,$$

where C_m is the membrane capacitance in $\mu f/cm^2$, and R_m is membrane resitivity in ohm-cm^2. The length constant indicates how the voltage decays along the fiber, neglecting time, whereas the time constant indicates how the voltage decays with time at any point. Thus a voltage at any point will decay to $1/e$ of its initial value in one time constant if there are no sources (applied voltages) present.

Conduction of an excitation along a nerve fiber depends on the core-conductor properties of the excitable fiber and on the ability of the membrane

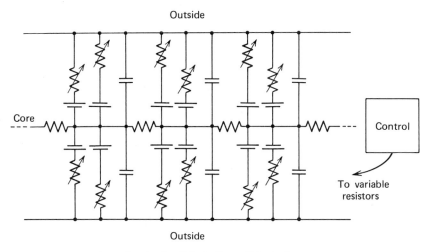

Figure 2.8 Equivalent circuit of cell including all batteries.

to develop a rapid change of potential by the mechanisms we have discussed. When a small area of a membrane is depolarized by the application of a stimulus the depolarization rapidly becomes regenerative, and the excited point reaches a different transmembrane potential from the rest of the unexcited fiber. The flow of current between excited and unexcited tissue is directed along the fiber by means of the conduction properties, so that the region next to the excited site is depolarized enough to become excited itself. As a result the excitation is conducted along the entire fiber. The depolarization itself is a result of the imbalance between sodium and potassium ions, which was initially discussed.

We can thus put together the two equivalent circuits we have been discussing into the composite of Figure 2.8. Figure 2.8 would correspond to a single cell, and a fiber would be made up of a number of these cells. The basic mechanism is now clear. A depolarization in a particular cell is represented by a shift in the values of the variable resistors in that cell. This presumably is initiated by an external stimulus of some kind. The stimulus is conducted to the adjacent cell by means of the conduction properties of the cell, which then cause the adjacent cell to depolarize. We have indicated this mechanism by a "control function" in Figure 2.8.

The time variation of the depolarization is of considerable interest, because the different fibers in the heart show different types of variations, which are understandable in mechanistic terms; for example, the waveform of the response of pacemaker cells from the S-A node are similar to what an

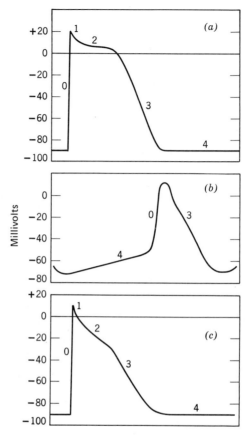

Figure 2.9   Transmembrane action potentials of various types of cardiac cells: (*a*) ventricle; (*b*) sinoatrial node; (*c*) atrium. (Modified from Hoffman and Cranefield [3]).

electrical engineer would expect to find from a free-running multivibrator whereas those from purely conductive cells are similar to the waveforms of a so-called "one-shot," or driven, multivibrator.

The transmembrane potentials of different cells in the heart exhibit various types of voltage variations. The potentials presented here are taken from Hoffman and Cranefield [3] and were measured by inserting a microelectrode into a cardiac cell and exciting the cell. The transmembrane potential was then recorded by using other microelectrodes. Although the shape and amplitude of the action potentials vary from one cell species to another and between fiber types, the action potentials from cardiac cells generally resemble those of other excitable cells in showing an initial rapid depolarization, or upstroke, but differ from the potentials of most other cells because they have a prolonged depolarization and a slow, delayed repolarization. The action potential of Figure 2.9 is typical of many ventricular cells: an initial rapid upstroke (phase 0), early rapid repolarization (phase 1), prolonged slow repolarization (phase 3), and the final diastolic period (phase 4). By contrast, an action potential from a spontaneously rhythmic pacemaker fiber is shown in Figure 2.9*b*. In the depolarization period of phase 4 the potential gradually rises instead of remaining constant. Eventually this potential reaches a threshold, which then results in excitation. Phases 1 and 2 are virtually indistinguishable, and at the end of phase 3 the cell is back to its initial condition, ready to start the cycle all over again.

The potential of Figure 2.9*c* is typical of those from most mammalian atrial fibers. Phase 2 of the repolarization is slow but not nearly so flat as it is in ventricular fibers—it actually can hardly be called a plateau. The period of initial rapid repolarization (phase 1) is sometimes absent.

As may be seen in Figure 2.9, the inside of the cell becomes positive with respect to the outside during the final phases of rapid repolarization as well as during the initial part of the period of repolarization. The amount of positive voltage is known as the overshoot and is ordinarily 15 to 20 mV in the fibers of the atrium and ventricle. It is greatly reduced or absent in the cells from the spontaneously rhythmic pacemaker (the S-A node). The overshoot is intimately related to the relative permeabilities of the cell to potassium and sodium ions, and is an important factor in determining the cell models that have been discussed previously.

The electrical activity of the heart may be observed as an electrocardiogram by electrodes on the skin surface. The components of the normal electrocardiogram are explained in Appendix C.

REFERENCES

[1] Heymans, C., and E. Neil, *Reflexogenic Areas of the Cardiovascular System,* Churchill, London, 1958.
[2] Rushmer, R. F., *Cardiovascular Dynamics,* Saunders, Philadelphia, 1961.
[3] Hoffman, B., and C. Cranefield, *Electrophysiology of the Heart,* McGraw-Hill, New York, 1960.
[4] Burton, A., *Physiology and Biophysics of the Circulation,* Year Book Medical Publishers, Chicago, 1965.
[5] Katz, B., *Nerve, Muscle, and Synapse,* McGraw-Hill, New York, 1966.

CHAPTER THREE

Blood Pressure Regulation

The mechanism by which the body regulates blood pressure is a complex feedback system that has been studied for a number of years. The advent of the carotid-sinus stimulator as a possible means of treating hypertension has lent new impetus to the physiology of this control system, since the electrical stimulation devices directly augment some of the organs involved. The general pattern of control is as follows: pressure-sensitive receptors (known as baroreceptors or pressoreceptors) located both at the carotid sinus in the neck and on the arch of the aorta detect mean and instantaneous blood pressure and transmit this information to the cardiac center in the medulla. From here impulses are sent to the heart and blood vessels to maintain the average blood pressure. In the normal subject the baroreceptors at the carotid sinus play a predominant part in blood-pressure regulation, and their role is the principal subject of this discussion.

Figure 3.1 shows the interrelation of pressure control and rate control in the body. A close relationship should be expected, since the basic purpose of the circulatory system is to supply adequate oxygen to the tissues by means of the circulating blood. The rate of perfusion depends on total blood delivered, which depends on pressure, flow, and rate. Thus these three quantities are all controlled simultaneously. Pressure and flow have their own set of interdependencies, since they are related to each other by the peripheral hydraulic resistance of the circulatory system, which is also under control of the central nervous system. In addition, the stroke volume of the heart is under some control (although the variation is not large in the normal subject).

The carotid sinus is located at the carotid "bulb," a dilation of the common carotid artery situated at its bifurcation below the angle or the jaw (Figure 3.2 shows the location of the artery). A nerve known as the carotid-sinus nerve (actually a branch of the ninth cranial nerve, the glossopharyngeal), runs from this region in the bifurcation formed by the internal and external carotid arteries. Although this structure and its nerve were known to the early anatomists, it was not realized that the sinus was a normal structure, or for that matter that it occurred normally. Similarly, the

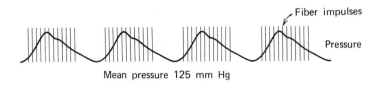

Mean pressure 125 mm Hg

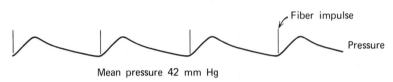

Mean pressure 42 mm Hg

Figure 3.1 Tracings showing that the carotid sinus activity depends both on absolute pressure and rate of change of pressure. (After Neil.)

anatomists of the last century regarded the nerve as only one of the many nerve twigs contributing to the intercarotid plexus. It was not until the 1920s that it was shown, principally by Hering and Heymans [1] that the carotid sinus was a reflexogenic area.

There are other baroreceptor areas in the common carotid artery, in addition to those at the sinus. Figure 3.2 shows their general location and in

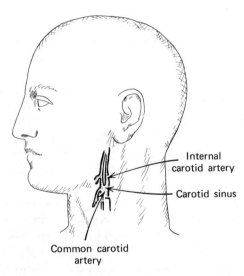

Figure 3.2 Sketch of the head showing the location of the carotid sinus.

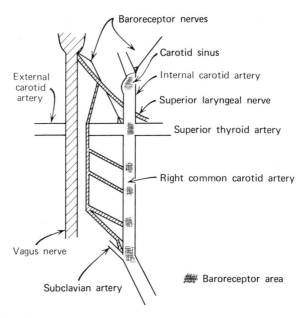

Figure 3.3   Location of various baroreceptor areas and a schematic representation of their anatomy.

addition gives some more detail of the anatomy (in a schematic fashion) of the carotid-sinus area.

The discovery of the depressor nerve in the neck by Cyon and Ludwig in 1886 first suggested the concept of reflex regulation of the cardiovascular system [1, 2]. Stimulating the peripheral end of the nerve produced bradycardia and hypertension. They were ignorant of the baroreceptors, believing that the depressor (aortic) nerve arose from endings in the heart itself, and they thought that the sensory endings were normally responsive to changes in intracardiac pressure. They thought that, if the heart beat too strongly, reflex bradycardia (abnormally slow heartbeat) or systemic hypotension (low blood pressure) would reduce the work of the heart. We now know that the aortic arch also contains baroreceptors and furthermore that these play a minor role in blood-pressure regulation.

The importance of the carotid sinus was not appreciated until 1923. It had been noticed as early as 1836 that occlusion of the common carotid arteries caused a rise of systemic blood pressure, and in 1866 it was reported that pressing firmly on the skin of the upper part of the neck (as we now know, this is over the carotid sinus) induced cardiac slowing; in general erroneous reasons were ascribed to these phenomena. One of the earliest attempts at this was Marey's law, which stated that a rise in blood pressure was usually associated with a slowing in pulse rate, and vice versa. There are many exceptions to this (e.g., both increase during exercise), so that it does not seem very useful as a generalization, although it is still included in some physiology courses [2, 3]. Hering made the actual discovery of the nature of the sinus because of his interest in cardiac slowing due to external pressure. In 1905, while performing this test on an old woman, he was struck by the fact that merely pressing lightly with the finger on one of her carotid arteries caused marked cardiac slowing. In 1923 he localized the origin of the reflex to nerve endings in the region of the carotid sinus, and in 1924 he proved that the excitation of the carotid-sinus wall in the dog caused not only reflex bradycardia but also reflex systemic hypotension. These effects were removed by cutting the carotid-sinus nerve. His experiments were particularly interesting because they summarized most of the external aspects of the reflex. An outline of these experiments is as follows [1, 2]:

1. A small clip placed on the carotid sinus in such a way that it caused mechanical stimulation but did not occlude the vessel completely produced slowing of the heart and a fall of blood pressure. Injection of atropine prevented the heart-slowing effect, although the hypotension still occurred, suggesting that there were two separate cardiovascular reflex responses.

2. Stimulation of the central end of the carotid-sinus nerve produced reflex bradycardia and hypotension.

3. Stretching (or pulling) the cephalic (upper) end of the common carotid artery produced the same response.

4. Introducing a probe into the cephalic end of the common carotid artery and stimulating the intimal wall of the sinus region induced the same reflex responses. These responses all could be prevented by cutting the sinus nerve.

5. Cutting both sinus nerves caused systemic hypertension.

Probably the most important studies of the carotid-sinus baroreceptors themselves were those conducted by Bronk and Stella in the early 1930s. They recorded nerve action potentials in the cut sinus nerve in rabbits, noting that a burst of action potentials occurred with each pulse. The nerve was then thinned by dissection, and in each of 25 experiments a single active nerve fiber was obtained. The single units fired with each systolic rise of pressure, the impulse frequency being greatest during the systolic upstroke of the pressure wave. The frequency of electrical impulses decreased as the blood pressure dropped from its peak, and in some cases the nerve stopped producing impulses at a higher pressure than the point at which they started during the upstroke. Bronk and Stella noted that when the impulses ceased during diastole at a certain pressure, and then the mean blood pressure was lowered by bleeding so that the peak systolic pressure was less than the previous diastolic pressure, the nerve then still produced action potentials during systole. From this experiment it became apparent that the response of the baroreceptor is not solely a function of the absolute level of blood pressure but includes other components and in particular depends on the rate of change of pressure.

More tests showed that the frequency of impulses from the sinus receptor is determined in large part by the rate of change of pressure. These effects can be seen in Figure 3.1, which shows that even at a mean pressure of 42 mm Hg the rise in systolic pressure may produce a single pulse, whereas in the first tracing there are no pulses during diastole, even though the mean pressure is 125 mm Hg.

Different baroreceptors were found to have different thresholds to both steady pressures and to the rate of change of pressure: higher pressure in the systemic circulation not only caused an increased frequency of discharge in a particular unit but also caused more units to fire. As the static pressure measured by an individual unit was changed, the frequency of impulses increased until a pressure level was reached at which the impulse frequency "saturated." Further increases in pressure did not produce corresponding increases in frequency. Below this range frequency and pressure were proportional. The saturation level varied with different receptors but was usually lower than 200 mm Hg. These points are illustrated in Figure 3.4, which shows the behavior of single units of the common carotid nerve. The electrical activity of the entire nerve, however, does not have such a systematic output but has very much the appearance of noise, with a detectable increase in activity, both in amplitude and frequency, during systolic periods. "Noise" here is used in a casual sense since the signals on the bundle are by no means chance events and, as has just been mentioned, the appearance of the action potentials changes with pressure. However, the signals picked up from the entire bundle do not have the neat characteristic of the frequency-modulated output of the single fiber, and visual inspection of the signal reveals little of their underlying character. The outputs from the individual receptors, on the other hand, exhibit regular changes in frequency with changes in pressure and rate of change of pressure, but no amplitude variations.

These experiments were all performed with isolated perfused carotid sinuses; that is, the arteries were isolated from the animals, and a pump or other external device was used to control the pressure measured by the baroreceptor. In effect the feedback loop was opened, and an external driving signal (a pressure in every case) was applied.

The general nature of the controls that have been discussed is shown in

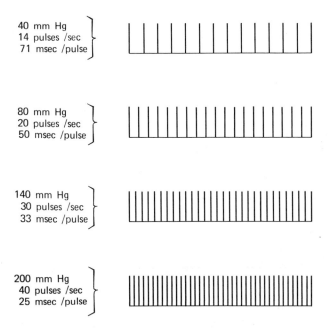

40 mm Hg
14 pulses /sec
71 msec /pulse

80 mm Hg
20 pulses /sec
50 msec /pulse

140 mm Hg
30 pulses /sec
33 msec /pulse

200 mm Hg
40 pulses /sec
25 msec /pulse

Figure 3.4   Behavior of single units of the carotid sinus pressure transducer. (After Bronk and Stella, *Am. J. Phys.* **110**:708, 1934.)

Figure 3.5. In order to show as many phenomena as possible, blood pressure and heart rate are indicated as having an inverse relationship although, as previously mentioned, this is not always true. The action potential on the sinoatrial nerve initiates each cardiac contraction. The rate of these impulses is controlled by the rate of impulses on the vagus nerve. Note that increased activity of the vagus nerve decreases the heart rate; thus the vagus nerve has an inhibiting action. The impulses on the carotid nerve follow the arterial pressure and its rate of change, the frequency of a single fiber being maximum where the rate of change of pressure is greatest (only the output of a single fiber is indicated for clarity). The sympathetic vasoconstrictor nerves call for increased vasoconstriction at low pressures, since greater peripheral resistance will tend to compensate for the loss in pressure [4].

The carotid-sinus stimulator does not represent an opening of the loop; it corresponds to an additional signal added to those already present. Some of the effects measured cannot be predicted directly from the data on perfused carotid sinuses. In particular, one does not observe the "all or none" reaction usually found in nerves and typical of the heart, which either beats or does not beat in response to an electrical stimulus. Work of the authors [5] in-

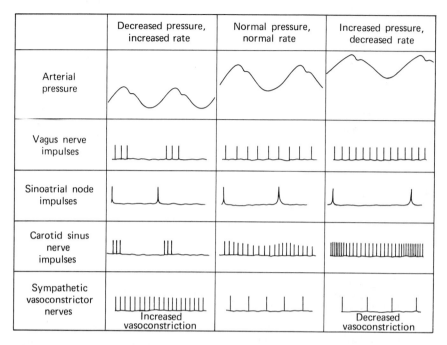

	Decreased pressure, increased rate	Normal pressure, normal rate	Increased pressure, decreased rate
Arterial pressure			
Vagus nerve impulses			
Sinoatrial node impulses			
Carotid sinus nerve impulses			
Sympathetic vasoconstrictor nerves	Increased vasoconstriction		Decreased vasoconstriction

Figure 3.5 Schematic illustration of responses and stimuli of various cardiac control reflexes. For simplicity, blood pressure and heart rate are shown as having inverse relationship (see text).

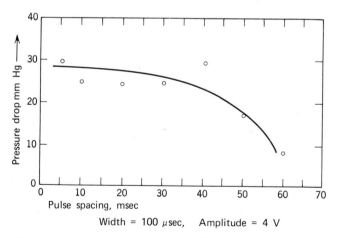

Width = 100 μsec, Amplitude = 4 V

Figure 3.6 Variation in blood pressure drop with carotid stimulator pulse spacing for a particular animal. This response was characteristic.

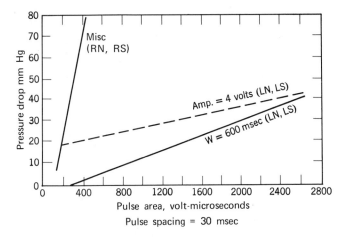

Figure 3.7 Pressure drop versus area of stimulating carotid-sinus pulse.

dicates that the drop in blood pressure seems to be approximately proportional to the area of an individual stimulating pulse (i.e., amplitude times duration) and to be relatively insensitive to the frequency of external stimulating pulses. Figure 3.6 shows the drop in blood pressure in a particular dog as a function of varying pulse frequency at a fixed amplitude and duration of the stimulating pulse. It can be seen that over a very wide range the drop in pressure does not depend on the frequency of the stimulating pulses. By comparison, Figure 3.7 shows the blood pressure drop plotted as a function of individual pulse area (i.e., energy per pulse) with pulse amplitude and width as parameters. It is apparent that the response depends on both amplitude and width, and as a first approximation is a function of only the product of these two quantities. However, for both width and amplitude there are stimulation thresholds below which the proportionality relations do not hold, and these thresholds seem to be separate, instead of there being one single threshold for energy. These proportionality constants and thresholds varied considerably from animal to animal, and between the left and right sides of the same animal, so these figures must be considered typical, rather than definitive.

The characteristics of the reflex as a servomechanism are of considerable interest, and in particular the transient response gives considerable information concerning the behavior of the control mechanism. The transient response can be determined by applying a constant stimulus and measuring its response until all transients die out, and then removing the stimulus, thus stimulating a step function. A typical result is shown in Figure 3.8. It can be seen that

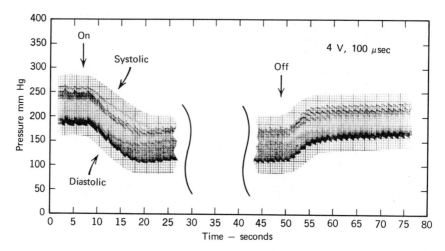

Figure 3.8 Transient response, showing blood pressure rise and fall when stimulus is suddenly applied and then removed.

the drop in pressure upon the application of the stimulus is noticeably slower than the rise in pressure upon its removal. Thus the carotid-sinus mechanism is at least time varying and is almost certainly nonlinear. The response times (about 25 sec for the pressure to decay to its steady-state value when the stimulus is applied and 10 sec to return to its initial value when the stimulus is removed) were, as well as could be determined, independent of the strength of the stimulus as long as the stimulus was within the "linear" range.

Tests were also made by the authors [5] to determine the effectiveness of stimulating both nerves, as contrasted to stimulating one at a time. It was found that, if both nerves were stimulated, the drop in pressure equalled the drop found with the most effective nerve; that is, if the left nerve produced a drop of 60 mm Hg and the right one 40 mm Hg when stimulated separately, the drop was 60 mm Hg when both were stimulated. In order to explore this effect further, one nerve was stimulated until the pressure drop had reached a plateau, and then the other nerve was cut. After a transient decrease lasting 15 to 20 sec, the pressure returned to the level it had before the nerve was cut. Precautions were taken to insure that these results were not dependent on the dissection techniques.

Early workers in the field observed cardiac slowing as well as drop in blood pressure upon electrical stimulation [1]. The work of the authors just presented indicates that the cardiac slowing does not seem to be caused by the stimulation on the baroreceptors themselves, but seems to be the result of the electrical stimulus' spreading to adjacent areas, perhaps to the vagus nerve, which lies nearby. With electrodes accurately placed so that there is no spread of electrical current, and with moderate stimuli, the only response observed is one of drop in blood pressure. With strong stimuli, however, changes both in heart rate and muscle twitching in the neck can be seen. Whether these are caused by the baroreceptors themselves at these high stimulation levels or are the result of stimulation of adjacent structures has not yet been determined.

REFERENCES

[1] Heymans, J. C., and E. Neil, *Reflexogenic Areas of the Cardiovascular System,* Churchill, London, 1958. Most of the historical material has been abstracted from this reference.
[2] Burton, A., *Physiology and Biophysics of the Circulation,* Year Book Medical Publishers, Chicago, 1965.
[3] Selkurt, E., *Physiology,* Little, Brown, Boston, 1963.
[4] Rushmer, R., *Cardiovascular Dynamics,* Saunders, Philadelphia, 1961.
[5] Myers, G., V. Parsonnet, G. Lewin, W. Holcomb, and I. Zucker. "Carotid Sinus Stimulus Parameters," *Med. Res. Eng.,* 7:13 (1968).

CHAPTER FOUR

Principles of Operation of Pacemakers

A cardiac pacemaker may be regarded as the electronic analog of a watch escapement. As a matter of fact, the basic concepts behind the construction of the two devices are similar in principle. The function of a watch escapement is to conserve the energy stored in the mainspring by releasing it when it is necessary to move the hands. In the same way, the electronic components of the pacemaker are designed to conserve the energy stored in the battery by dissipating it only when it is necessary to stimulate the heart. The energy called for from the mainspring and from the battery during the quiescent periods of the two devices is negligible; as a matter of fact, these devices use very little energy during the time they are operating.

The regulation of the frequency of a watch (the time interval between beats) is determined by the inertia of the balance wheel and its associated spring. The basic concept behind the operation of the balance wheel is that a small amount of energy is first stored in the spring, which is then released at a controlled rate that depends only on the physical constants of the system (the stiffness of the spring and the shape of the wheel), and not on the total amount of energy remaining in the mainspring. A subsidiary concept is that a small amount of stored energy in the balance-wheel spring controls a large amount of stored energy in the mainspring. It is the presence of the escapement and balance wheel that distinguish a watch from the familiar wind-up-spring toys, which actually store much more energy in their springs than does a watch. Thus the speed of a spring toy depends on how much the mainspring is wound up.

The frequency-regulating principle of the pacemaker also depends on energy storage, but in this case the storage device is the electrical capacitor. The principles of the electric circuit elements, for those unfamiliar with them, are discussed in Appendix A. Briefly, if C is the value of the capacitor (measured in farads), and Q is the amount of charge stored in it (measured in coulombs), then the voltage V appearing across the terminals of the capacitor is given by the formula $Q = CV$.

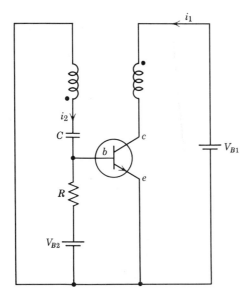

Figure 4.1 Schematic diagram of a blocking oscillator circuit.

The energy stored in the capacitor is released into a resistor. If R is the value of the resistor in ohms, then the time required to dissipate approximately 63 percent of the charge stored in the capacitor is given by the quantity RC, whose dimensions are in seconds. Thus the numerical value of this product is a measure of the amount of time for the charge to be dissipated. From the formula relating the charge to the voltage it can be seen that if there is no charge stored in the condenser, there is no voltage across it; thus by monitoring the voltage across the capacitor we can measure time. It is important to note that the time required to discharge the capacitor does not depend on the amount of charge stored in it, so that this time constant is suitable for a time standard. To return to the analogy, the time required for one swing of a pendulum does not depend in any critical way on the initial deflection of the wheel or pendulum (i.e., on the amount of energy initially stored in it).

Most (although not all) pacemakers are of the form of electronic circuit known as a blocking oscillator, one form of which is illustrated in Figure 4.1.* The circuit shown is similar to one used in the Medtronic pacemakers.† The figure shows an *npn* transistor, but a *pnp* could have been used

---

* The reader unfamiliar with circuit notation is urged to read Appendix A before this chapter.

† Medtronic Corp., Minneapolis, Minn.

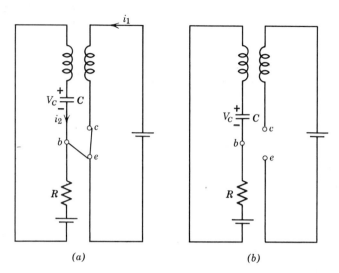

Figure 4.2   A blocking oscillator with a transistor either conducting or not conducting:
(*a*) transistor conducting; (*b*) transistor not conducting.

just as well if the battery voltages were reversed. This circuit can be
explained by using the approximation that the transistor acts like a voltage-
controlled switch. When the circuit is first turned on the full battery voltage of V_{B2} is applied to the base of the transistor, causing it to conduct as
shown in Figure 4.2*a*. The collector current i_1 goes into a dot on the primary side of the transformer and comes out of the dot on the secondary as
i_2. This current finds a low-resistance path from base to emitter, and so
almost all of it flows by this route, which tends to keep the transistor conducting (i.e., the current i_2 flowing from base to emitter is in the same direction as the current from the battery V_{B2} flowing in that branch, and so
aids the battery in keeping the transistor on). However, this same current
i_2 is charging the capacitor C with the polarity indicated, the terminal next
to the base becoming negative. Eventually the capacitor charges to a sufficiently high voltage for the base terminal to become negative with respect
to the emitter (this happens when the voltage across the capacitor becomes
greater than V_{B2}), and the transistor then turns itself off, as shown in Figure 4.2*b*. The transistor is now virtually an open circuit, and the capacitor
will discharge through the resistor R. As was just discussed, the time it takes
for the capacitor to discharge is proportional to the product (time constant)
RC. When the capacitor has discharged enough for the base again to become
positive the transistor starts conducting again, and the whole cycle repeats.

The time between pulses (slightly less than 1 sec for a cardiac pacemaker) is thus governed by the values of the resistor R and the capacitor C.

The duration of the pulse is the time during which the transistor is conducting. If the transformer were truly an ideal transformer and the transistor truly a short-circuit when it conducts, then the pulse duration would be infinitely short, because the capacitor C would charge up instantly and then immediately turn the transistor "off." Of course, this is not true. The transistor actually has a certain amount of resistance when it is conducting, whereas the transformer, which is made of wire, has both resistance and inductance. It is basically the resistance and inductance of the transformer that supplies a time constant during the charging of the capacitor C and thus controls the width of the pulse. A certain amount of time is required for current to start flowing in the windings of the transformer. This time interval controls the pulse width. If a different pulse width is desired, it is usually necessary to design a new transformer.

The blocking oscillator is an excellent time regulator but, like the watch escapement, cannot provide much power to the outside world. If we were to try to take much power from the transistor, we would find that the timing relations would be upset, because taking power is equivalent to adding resistance, and the timing relations all depend on the resistance present. This would be especially difficult in a pacemaker, because the "load" (the tissue being stimulated) has a resistance R_4 (impedance) which varies with time, so that the interval between pulses would be unpredictable. Because of this practical pacemakers use a second transistor as an amplifier.

One way of accomplishing this is shown in Figure 4.3. A third winding has been added to the transformer, which is connected to the base of a second transistor. This transistor is normally kept nonconducting by the negative voltage of V_{B3}, but the pulse in the transformer caused by the conduction of the blocking oscillator causes the second transistor to conduct also. During the period in which the second transistor (Q_2) has been nonconducting, the capacitor C_2 has charged up to voltage V_{B1} through R_2 with the time constant R_2C_2. Resistor R_2 is made as large as possible, so as little current as possible flows through the heart, because all of the charging current must flow through the heart. The time constant in this interval is actually $(R_2 + R_H)C_2$, but the resistance of the heart, R_H, is negligible compared with R_2. When transistor Q_2 conducts the capacitor is virtually placed right across the heart (because the transistor is now a short circuit), and the heart receives a pulse equal in amplitude to V_{B1}. The capacitor will discharge during this interval with a time constant equal to R_HC_2, and this discharge can actually be observed with many pacemakers. Usually capacitor C_2 is made so large that the decay is not appreciable. When the transistor be-

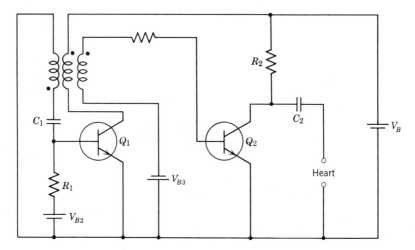

Figure 4.3 A practical pacemaker circuit using a blocking oscillator and an output amplifier.

comes nonconducting resistor R_2 is placed in series with the load, and the current drops to a very low value.

Thus the second transistor acts as a valve. A very small amount of power at its input (the base) can control a much greater amount of power at its output. Furthermore, its characteristics are relatively stable, so that any effects of the amplifier circuit on the blocking oscillator itself can be compensated for in the initial design. Changes in heart resistance have almost no effect on the amplifier circuit, the principal one being a change in discharge rate of capacitor C_2, which is small under any circumstances.

In the example shown a fixed voltage was used for pacing; that is, the capacitor was charged to a fixed voltage during the "off" time of the transistor. During the stimulation period the current in the load is $I_L = V_C/R_H$, where V_C is the voltage to which the capacitor has been charged. Changes in the load R_H will not affect V_C in this circuit, but clearly change the current flowing during the stimulation period.

It is believed that in many clinical applications the current rather than the voltage should be constant during the stimulation period because, physiologically, the current appears to be the factor that actually causes a response [1]. This is discussed in more detail later. One possible way of acquiring a constant current is shown in Figure 4.4, which is a schematic drawing of the voltage stimulator just described. The battery with voltage V corresponds to the charged capacitor, and the switch corresponds to the transistor. Whenever the switch closes, the battery is connected across the

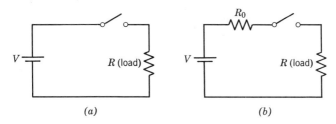

Figure 4.4 An ideal voltage source and a physical source: (*a*) ideal; (*b*) physical.

load R, and a current (given by Ohm's law) of $I = V/R$ flows. Now suppose a large resistor of value R_0 is placed in series with the battery, where R_0 is much greater than the maximum value of the load resistor R. The current will then be $I = V/(R + R_0)$. If R_0 is enough bigger than R (say by a factor of 10), then the actual value of the current will be almost independent of the exact value of the load resistor R and will in fact by almost equal to V/R_0. Of course, if the same current is desired in this second case as in the first case, the voltage V must be increased (by a factor of 10 if R_0 is 10 times as large as R).

For an implanted pacemaker it is usually impractical to make R_o and V large enough to make the current entirely independent of the load. For most pacing applications a current of approximately 2 ma is required during the pulse, and the load resistance varies from about 300 to 1000 ohms. Thus, if a 10,000-ohm series resistor were used for R_0, then the battery voltage would have to be about 30 volts to supply the required current. Because such a large battery is impractical in an implanted unit, so-called current-source pacemakers are usually compromises—there is some resistance in series with the load, but usually not enough to make the current truly independent of the load resistance.

A generator that delivers a current independent of the load resistance is called a current source; one that delivers a voltage independent of the load resistance is called a voltage source. As has been shown, one way of approximating a current source is to connect a large resistance in series with a voltage source and a load. Actually, true voltage sources and true current sources do not exist, but the common battery is a goood approximation to a true voltage source. In pacemaker applications current sources are usually constructed as indicated; that is, a series resistor and a high-voltage battery. In other applications, however, there are alternative methods for obtaining a current source. Certain transistors (not the switching transistors used in pacemaker circuits) and certain electronic tubes do approximate current sources over a limited range of output currents. It is also possible to con-

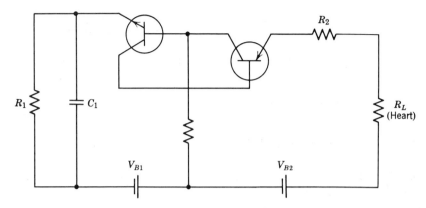

Figure 4.5   A pacemaker circuit using a multivibrator made from a *pnp* and an *npn* transistor.

struct fairly complex circuits that will hold currents very nearly constant, but these usually have too many components to be useful for implanted devices.

Another circuit often employed [2] in pacemakers is shown in Figure 4.5. Note that this uses a combination of an *npn* and a *pnp* transistor, and has no transformer. The connection of the transistors is such that if one conducts, both conduct. When the circuit is first turned on, the positive voltage of V_{B1} causes the two transistors to become conductive. Capacitor C_1 then charges up. Typically R_1 is much greater than R_2 or the load resistor R_L, so capacitor C_1 basically has the two batteries, V_{B1} and V_{B2} connected across its terminals. If this condition were maintained long enough, C_1 would eventually charge up to the voltage $(V_{B1} + V_{B2})$ with a time constant given by $(R_2 + R_L)C_1$. But once the voltage across C_1 becomes greater than V_{B1} the transistors will become nonconducting. Capacitor C_1 will then discharge through resistor R_1. When it is sufficiently discharged the transistors will conduct again, and the cycle will repeat.

The interval between pulses is controlled by the time constant R_1C_1, whereas the pulse width is controlled by the time constant $(R_2 + R_L)C_1$. If R_2 is made much larger than R_L, then the pulse width is independent of the load resistor. However, an interesting situation occurs if R_2 is made much smaller than R_L; in this case the pulse width will be proportional to the load resistor R_L. The energy dissipated in the load for any of these circuits is V^2W/R_L, where W is the pulse width. If the pulse width W is proportional to R_L, then R_L cancels out. Note that the voltage appearing across the load $(V_{B1} + V_{B2})$, which corresponds to V in the energy equa-

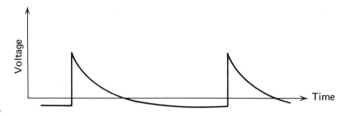

Figure 4.6 Exponential waveform found with some pacemakers.

tion, does not depend on the load resistor. The capacitor will always charge to the same voltage independent of the load. Thus if R_2 is much smaller than R_L, the energy dissipated in the load on each pulse is given approximately by $\frac{1}{2} V^2 C_1$ and is independent of the load resistance. For this reason this circuit is often referred to as a constant-energy, or constant-power, pacemaker.

The pulse width has been discussed for the above two circuits as if the output pulses were identical for the two. This is not actually the case. In the constant-energy circuit just discussed the output pulse follows the charge current of the capacitor C and has the appearance shown in Figure 4.6. The sudden rise in voltage corresponds to the time when the transistors start conducting, and the exponential drop corresponds to the gradual decrease in current as the capacitor charges up. The discharge current, which occurs during the interpulse period, is negligible.

The blocking oscillator, on the other hand, has an almost rectangular pulse, as shown in Figure 4.7. If it is a voltage source, this will be the voltage waveform; whereas if it is a current source, it will be the current waveform. The slight "droop" on the top of the pulse is caused by the slight discharge of the capacitor C_2 in Figure 4.3. If the load is a true resistance, the waveforms of both current and voltage will look like those in the figures, independent of whether the source is a voltage or a current source. However, the load is not resistive because of polarization effects, which are discussed in a later chapter. Thus current and voltage waveforms are not identical.

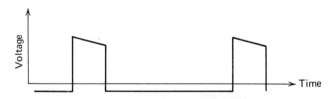

Figure 4.7 Rectangular waveform found with most makes of pacemaker.

FIGURE 4.8

Manufacturer	Model	Type	Commercially Available	Fixed Rate	Variable Rate	Maximum Energy Output (μJ)	Output Current (ma) [Test Load (ohms)]
Airborne Instruments, Deer Park, N.Y.	496-1 497-2	A,R	NO		40 to 120	405	5-45 [200]
Cordis Corp., Miami, Fla.	Ventricor	A	YES	60-90	NO		
	Demand	A,D	NO	70	NO	130	10 [500]
	Atricor	S	YES		65-125		
Electrodyne, Norwood, Mass.	TR14	A	YES	70	NO	196	14 [500]
General Electric, Milwaukee, Wis.	A2072BA	A	YES	70	NO	70	20 [300]
	A2072AA	A	YES		70 or 85		
	A2070BA	A	YES	70		50	12.5 [300]
	A2070AA	A	YES		70 or 85		
Medtronic, Minneapolis, Minn.	5859	A	YES	55-120	NO	45	3 or 5 [1000]
	5859C	A	YES				
	5860	A	YES	55-120	NO	80	3.5 or 6.5 [1000]
	5860C	A	YES				7 [1000]
	5864	A	YES	55-120	NO	60	0-6 [1000]
	5864C	A	YES			50	0-5.5 [1000]
	5870	A	YES	55-120		60	0-6 [1000]
	5870C	A	YES			50	0-5.5 [1000]
	5841	D	NO	55-100		63	6 [1000]

A = Asynchronous
B = Bipolar
U = Unipolar
BI = Biphasic
BP = Back Plate of Pulse Generator

Figure 4.8 Chart showing current status of American-manufactured pacemaker (modified from Judson, Glenn and Holcomb, "Cardiac Pacemakers," *J. Surg. Res.* **7**:527 (1967).

FIGURE 4.8 (*continued*)

Manufacturer	Output Voltage (V) [Test Load (ohms)]	Wave-form	Pulse Dura-tion (msec)	Area (cm²)	Height (cm)	Weight (gm)	Elec-trodes
Airborne Instruments, Deer Park, N.Y.	1-9 [200]	M BI	1.0	10.0	0.75	25	UM BI
Cordis Corp., Miami, Fla.	6.5 [∞]	BI	1.8-2.0	24.5	2.2	130	UB,UM UB,UM UM
Electrodyne, Norwood, Mass.	7.0 [∞]	BI	2.0	46.0	2.0	180	BM
General Electric, Milwaukee, Wis.	6.0 [∞]	BI	2.5	31.0	2.0	140	BM
	3.7 [∞]	BI	2.5	31.0	2.0	120	BE
Medtronic, Minneapolis, Minn.	3 or 5 [1000]	BI	1.75	28.5	1.8	130	BM BE
	3.5 or 6.5 [1000] 5.5 [1000]	BI	1.75	31.0 28.5	2.5 2.5	200	BM BE
	0-5.5 [1000] 0-4.5 [1000]	BI	1.75	31.0 28.5	2.5 2.5	200	BM BE
	0-5.5 [1000] 0-4.5 [1000]	BI	1.75	31.0 28.5	2.5 2.5	200	BM BE
	6 [1000]	BI	1.75	28.5	2.5	200	BE

D/S = Demand (or stand by)
EL = Elgiloy
E = Transvenous Endocardial
M = Transthoracic Myocardial
R = Radio Coupled

The basic principles of stimulator circuit construction are similar, whether it is designed for the heart, carotid sinus, or other. However, the actual stimuli supplied to the load are different. For a cardiac pacemaker the rate is between one and two pulses per second, whereas for a carotid-sinus pacemaker it is about 30 to 60 pulses per second. The amplitudes and widths also vary. The descriptions of these circuits have indicated how these various parameters may be controlled. The table in Figure 4.8 gives the ranges of values used in different pacing applications today.

So far the discussion has been devoted exclusively to the implanted asynchronous pacemaker because it is the most fundamental of the various pacemaker circuits. There are several important modifications of this basic circuit to be discussed:

1. The synchronous pacemaker.
2. The radio-frequency-energized (or RF) pacemaker.
3. The standby pacemaker.

It is not necessary to distinguish between the precise applications of these devices, since in general the waveform of the output voltage or current can be varied at will by means of relatively minor circuit variations. Note that both current *and* voltage cannot be changed arbitrarily; for example, if current is regulated, the voltage will be determined by the impedance of the electrodes and tissues. The nature of this impedance is discussed later. The discussion here emphasizes the basic principles of the various devices.

The asynchronous pacemaker has a rate that is independent of any physiological variable. The synchronous pacemaker is intended to improve body function by causing the heart to beat at its natural rate, as determined by the sinoatrial node. A block diagram of a commonly used synchronous pacer is shown in Figure 4.9 [3]. In this pacemaker an extra electrode is fastened to the atrium, where the P wave is detected, and is then amplified. A transmission delay of 0.16 sec is now necessary, corresponding to the actual delay in conducting the P wave to the atrioventricular node in the normal heart. The signal is then used to control an amplifier, which produces the desired stimulus to be applied to the heart. With this type of pacemaker certain safety features must be incorporated. If the rate of atrial excitation becomes too fast (as in atrial fibrillation) or too slow, a preset fixed rate must take over until the abnormal situation is over. This has been accomplished by having an asynchronous pacer set to operate at the slowest desired rate, approximately 55 per minute in many cases. If a signal from the amplified P wave is applied to one of the "off" transistors in the oscillator circuit, it will cause it to fire before the next anticipated fixed pulse. If no natural P wave occurs, the pacemaker will produce a pulse at a preset delay from its previous stimulus.

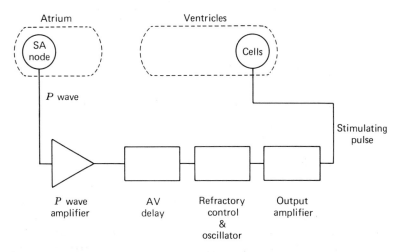

Figure 4.9 Block diagram of synchronous pacemaker.

A maximum rate (115 to 120 per minute in one type) is also included and is controlled by a blocking circuit, so that the output pulse will be one-half the signal rate or one-third its rate if the signal is greater than 180 per minute.

Normally the pacemaker pulse is so large that it would be detected by the atrial pickup lead and cause the heart to beat. This problem has been eliminated by building in a "refractory" period (i.e., any signal detected on the atrial lead within 400 msec of a paced heartbeat is ignored).

In some clinical situations heart block may be intermittent. Thus, if a pacemaker is implanted in such a patient, the artificial pacemaker at such times would be unnecessary, and the patient will then have two pacemakers, his own natural one and the implanted one as well. If a stimulus falls in the vulnerable period, ventricular fibrillation may result. To solve this problem the standby pacemaker has been developed. In a way, the standby pacemaker may be considered to be the inverse of the synchronous pacer, and indeed the circuitry is basically a modification of that used in the synchronous application. In the standby pacer the heart rate is detected—but should it fall below a certain minimum level, an asynchronous pacer is turned on to pace the heart. A block diagram of this device is shown in Figure 4.10. The lead used to stimulate the heart is also used to detect the R wave, which is the signal that the ventricles have contracted. The R wave is amplified and is applied to a blocking circuit. If a natural contraction occurs, the asynchronous pacer's timing circuit is reset so that it will time its next pulse from the detected heartbeat. Otherwise the asynchronous pacer produces

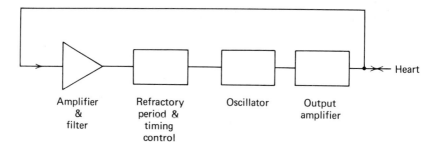

Figure 4.10 Block diagram of standby pacemaker.

pulses at its preset rate. One way of achieving this, for example, is to discharge the timing capacitor in one of the pacemaker circuits just indicated.

Certain special safety features are built into this circuit. The pacemaker, for example, might detect "noise" and interpret it as a ventricular excitation. This problem has been solved, as in the synchronous pacer, by incorporating a refractory period after either a natural or paced contraction. Signals detected immediately after the contraction are ignored. A more serious problem is inadvertent pickup of other electrocardiographic waves. The *P* waves may, for example, be quite large when measured either on the surface, or in the interior, of the ventricle. A refractory period cannot help here, since *P* waves occur at random times with respect to ventricular excitations in heart block. Fortunately, the *P* and *R* waves have their principal energy in different frequency bands. A high-pass filter with a lower cutoff frequency of 20 Hz almost completely eliminates the *P* wave. The *R* wave is differentiated by such a filter, and its peak-to-peak amplitude is increased [4].

From a physiological point of view the synchronous and standby pacemakers are far superior to the fixed-rate pacemakers. However, they obtain their advantages by a considerable increase in complexity. A synchronous pacemaker may have more than 32 parts, including more than six transistors, as compared with approximately eight components (including the two transistors) in the fixed-rate model. The extra transistors dissipate power, and consequently the battery life of the synchronous and standby pacers is shorter. In the case of the standby pacemaker the effect on battery life is counterbalanced by the fact that relatively little power is dissipated when the heart rate is normal, which increases the life expectancy of the units. Whether the additional complexity and shorter life of these devices overcome their advantages is a judgment each physician must make. Experience with these units, however, has been very good, and premature failures are rare.

It is possible to construct a standby pacemaker by modifying a synchronous pacemaker. In the synchronous pacemaker one of the safety features is a timing circuit that produces an output pulse if no P wave has been detected. To make a standby pacemaker only two electrodes are used, and the R wave is detected instead of the P wave. The timing circuit is adjusted so that, if an R wave is present, the pacemaker will produce a stimulus immediately after the R wave. The stimulus will then occur in the refractory period of the cardiac cycle, a time when electrical stimuli produce no excitation or mechanical response in the ventricles. Otherwise the pacemaker will produce a pulse a fixed time after the preceding output stimulus, as in a regular pacemaker. This premature firing may be easily accomplished by having the R-wave discharge the timing capacitor through an additional transistor. An advantage of this method is that the pacemaker is always producing pulses (even though many occur during periods when they are ineffective because the natural rhythm is present), and thus an electrocardiogram will always show whether the pacemaker is working. With the other type of standby pacemaker no output stimuli are present during normal rhythm, and thus it is difficult to determine whether the batteries or any other component have failed.

The radio-frequency-energized pacemaker is intended to overcome some of the finite battery life problems of an implanted pacemaker [5, 6, 7]. In these devices almost all of the electronics are worn externally. Implanted inside the body are a small receiving antenna and passive detection circuits (i.e., no devices such as transistors, which require batteries). Two different principles have been employed in the design of these devices. In both an asynchronous pacer of the type previously discussed forms the basic element. In one of these the output amplifier is connected directly to a coil that is placed next to the chest wall. Another coil is placed just opposite it under the skin of the chest wall. Energy is transferred by electromagnetic induction, and no radio-frequency energy is used; the two coils act as the primary and secondary of a pulse transformer, so that the pulse going into the primary on the outside of the chest is picked up by the secondary winding on the inside, much as is done by the transformer in the blocking oscillator just discussed. However, because the windings cannot be placed very close to each other, and as a matter of fact are separated by a conducting medium (the skin and blood, and related tissue) losses are very high, and very large power must be supplied by the external device. As a result the battery life is short, and, even though the batteries are external, they require replacement every few weeks. No surgical procedure is involved, however.

A more efficient alternative is to use a carrier, as shown in the circuit block diagram in Figure 4.11. A blocking oscillator generates pulses just as

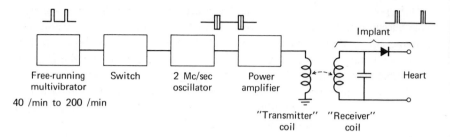

Figure 4.11 Block diagram of radio-frequency energized pacemaker.

in an ordinary implanted pacemaker, but now these pulses are used to turn on a 2 MHz oscillator instead of stimulating the heart. The high-frequency oscillations are amplified in a power amplifier and transmitted into the body by means of a transmitter coil. The condenser and rectifier connected to the receiving coil beneath the skin remove the 2 MHz carrier, and a transformer is then used to remove the direct-current component developed by the recti-

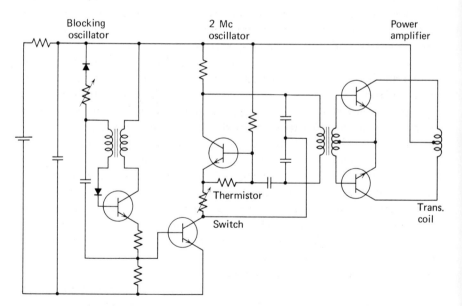

Figure 4.12 Schematic diagram of radio-frequency pacemaker.

fier. Because of the increased efficiency realized by transmitting at a frequency of 2 MHz, this device can be built with batteries that last from 6 months to a year. An actual circuit of one type of pacemaker is shown in Figure 4.12.

REFERENCES

[1] Furman, S., B. Parker, and D. Escher, "Endocardial Electrical Threshold of Human Cardiac Response as a Function of Surface Area," *Dig. 7th Int. Conf. Med. and Biol. Eng.*, 1967, p. 71.

[2] Kantrowitz, A., R. Cohen, H. Raillard, J. Schmidt, and D. Feldman, "The Treatment of Complete Heart Block with an Implanted, Controllable Pacemaker," *Surg. Gynec. Obstet.*, 115:415 (1962).

[3] Nathan, D., S. Center, P. Samet, C. Y. Wu, and J. Keller, "The Application of Implantable Synchronous Pacer for the Correction of Stokes-Adams Attacks," *Ann. N. Y. Acad. Sci.*, 111:1093 (1964).

[4] Parsonnet, V., I. R. Zucker, L. Gilbert, and G. H. Myers, "Clinical Use of an Implantable Standby Pacemaker," *JAMA*, 196:784 (1966).

[5] Widmann, W., W. Glenn, L. Eisenberg, and A. Mauro, "Radio-Frequency Cardiac Pacemaker," *Ann. N. Y. Acad. Sci.*, 111:992 (1964).

[6] Camilli, L., R. Pozzi, G. Pizzichi, and G. De Saint-Pierre, "Radio-Frequency Pacemaker with Receiver Coil Implanted in the Heart," ibid., 1007.

[7] Abrams, L., and J. Norman, "Experience with Inductive Coupled Cardiac Pacemakers," ibid., 1030.

CHAPTER FIVE

Theoretical Prediction of Pacemaker Stimulus Thresholds

1. INTRODUCTION

In order to optimize the design of a pacemaker it is important to be able to analyze theoretically the interface between the electrode and the cardiac tissue, so that the important factors affecting stimulation may be properly recognized. This chapter presents a theory that may be used to derive pacing thresholds for common shapes of pacemaker electrodes and to analyze other tissue stimulators. The theory agrees quantitatively with the experimental results of a number of other investigators [1–5], although most of the experimental work presented in the literature has not included enough detail for direct comparisons with the analysis presented here. As a result some experimental data collected by the authors that are more applicable to the theory are also presented. The theory itself makes many approximations and simplifications to the complex problem of tissue stimulation and the phenomena occurring in cells when they depolarize. However, it does permit the approximate calculation of stimulation thresholds and it indicates the relationships between the various electrode and cell parameters that affect the thresholds.

The basis for much of the work presented here was suggested by Lale [6], Katz [7], and Loewenstein [8]. These references, as well as Hoffman and Cranefield [1], may be consulted for additional material on relevant electrophysiology.

All effects of electrode polarization are neglected in this chapter. In effect an "ideal" electrode is assumed. The characteristics of physical electrodes, and their effects on stimulation, are discussed in the next chapter.

The following results are presented in this chapter:

1. A method for computing thresholds for stimuli of long duration ("rheobase") for electrodes of spherical and cylindrical shapes is derived.

2. A method for computing strength-duration curves is derived. It is shown that there is an optimum pulse width if minimum energy is to be supplied by the pacemaker, which is related to the membrane resistance and capacitance of the individual cells.

3. Characteristics of surface electrodes are derived.

It is assumed that there are electrically excitable cells in the immediate vicinity of the electrodes and that the excitation spreads over the myocardium if any single cell depolarizes. A transmission line model of the cell is used, in which the cell has a membrane resistance (unit: ohm $=$ cm^2) and capacitance (unit: farad/cm^2) and a longitudinal resistance in its inner core (unit: ohm-cm). A model of the cell is shown in Figure 5.1; for convenience it is assumed that the cell lies along the x-axis. By applying standard transmission line techniques it can be shown [6] that the equations relating current and voltage along the cell are

$$\frac{\partial v}{\partial x} = \frac{\rho}{A} i,$$

$$\frac{\partial i}{\partial x} = 2xr_c \left[\frac{V - v}{R_m} + c \frac{d}{dt} (V - v) \right] \qquad \lambda^2 = \frac{R_m r_c}{2\rho}, \qquad (1)$$

where $V =$ the potential of the external medium at x,

$R_m =$ the resistance of 1 cm^2 of membrane,

$c =$ the capacitance of 1 cm^2 of membrane,

$r_c =$ the radius of the cell,

$i =$ the current flowing through the inner core,

$v =$ the voltage in the inner core at x,

$\rho =$ the resistivity of the inner core,

$A =$ the cross-sectional area of the inner core,

$\lambda =$ the characteristic length of the cell (the length such that the radial resistance of that length of membrane equals the longitudinal resistance of that length of inner core).

End effects in the cells are neglected.

The purpose of the implanted electrode is to set up an electric field in the cardiac tissue (assumed to be a homogeneous conducting medium). If the potential difference across the membrane ($V - v$) exceeds some critical threshold value in any one cell, that cell will depolarize. The depolarization of any one cell will in turn cause adjacent cells to depolarize, with the re-

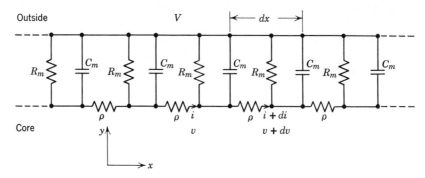

Figure 5.1 Equivalent circuit of cell, showing transmission line model. *Note.* Resistances and capacitances per unit length and area have been indicated for clarity. Actually these quantities should be $\rho \, dx$, R_m/dA, and so on.

sult that in a short time the depolarization will spread over the entire myocardium. In general this depolarization wave will cause both ventricles to contract (or the atria if the stimulus is applied there). This critical value of $V - v$, called V_T, is on the order of 50 mV [1].

In Section 2, the effects of capacitance are neglected. The thresholds computed in this way are those that would apply when a very long stimulating pulse is used (this concept is made more explicit later) and are often known as the rheobase. The effects of capacitance will then be considered by an approximate method in Section 5.

2. RHEOBASE THRESHOLDS OF IMPLANTED SPHERES AND CYLINDERS

If the effects of capacitance are neglected, then (1) may be simplified to

$$(v - V) = \lambda^2 \frac{d^2v}{dx^2} = \frac{R_m}{2r_c} \frac{di}{dx}, \tag{2}$$

where the total derivative may be used, since there is no time variation. Lale [6] points out that this may be approximated by replacing d^2v/dx^2 by d^2V/dx^2; that is, by using the potential in the medium in place of the potential in the core. This equivalency for $r >> \lambda$ is proved in Appendix B. In addition, Lale presents numerical computations to justify the result. The agreement of this theory with experiments discussed in Section 6 is close enough to provide additional confidence in the validity of the assumption. Therefore this approximation is used in the development that follows.

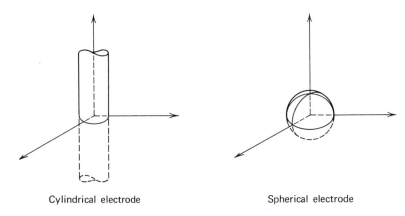

Cylindrical electrode   Spherical electrode

Figure 5.2   Electrode geometry used for theoretical calculations.

The assumed electrode geometry is shown in Figure 5.2. The centers of the cylindrical electrodes lie at the origin, with the axis of the cylinder lying along the z-axis. Spherical electrodes also have their center at the origin. In both cases the other (indifferent) electrode is assumed to lie at infinity. For the cylindrical electrode end effects are neglected. Therefore the theory applies to long, thin cylinders. No current flows from the ends. In the experiments to be cited later this condition is met by insulating both ends of the cylinder so that the electrode itself is basically a bare section of an insulated wire. The pacemaker source is assumed to be a current source with a total current I passing through the electrode.

The procedure used in the derivation is as follows: The current density in the tissue is computed from the known boundary conditions and the facts that the electrodes are at a uniform potential (because they are perfect conductors) and have a uniform current density at the interface between the electrode and tissue (because of symmetry). The current density in the medium can then be computed. From this the total current and its gradient are calculated. The gradient is then related to the transmembrane potential by means of (2), which permits computation of the thresholds.

A.   *Cylindrical Electrode*

The electrode is assumed to be of length e and radius a. If the total current into the electrode is I, then this current will pass through all cylinders of tissue concentric with the electrode, and the current density j, which must be independent of θ, in any transverse plane (plane parallel to the x-y plane) is given by

$$j(r) = \frac{I}{2\pi rl} \mathbf{u}_r, \tag{3}$$

where r is radial distance from the origin and $\mathbf{u}_r$ is the unit vector in the radial direction. It can be shown that the maximum gradient of current is in the radial direction. If a cell of cross-sectional area A lies along a radius, then the current through the cell is given by

$$i(r) = j \cdot \mathbf{A} = \frac{I}{2\pi rl} A. \tag{4}$$

The derivative of current with respect to radius (all current flows in the radial direction from symmetry) is then

$$\frac{di}{dr} = -\frac{IA}{2\pi lr^2}. \tag{5}$$

By using (2) and replacing (d^2v/dr^2) by (d^2V/dr^2), we obtain

$$v - V = \frac{\lambda^2 IA}{2\pi lr^2}. \tag{6}$$

At threshold $v - V = V_T$ and $I = -I_0$ (reflecting the well-known fact that stimulation takes place at the cathode). Thus the threshold current is given by

$$I_0 = \frac{V_T}{\rho\lambda^2} (2\pi lr^2), \tag{7}$$

where the definition of λ has been used to simplify (7). In (7) r is the distance from the electrode of the nearest sensitive tissue. Since the threshold is lowest for small r and there is probably a sensitive cell near the electrode, r may be replaced by a, the electrode radius. Thus the formula for the threshold current reduces to

$$I_0 = \frac{2V_T}{\rho\lambda^2} (\pi la^2) \tag{8}$$

for cylindrical electrodes. Note that the quantity in parentheses is the volume of the electrode.

B. Spherical Electrode

The development for the spherical electrode follows exactly the same lines as for the cylindrical electrode, except now the current density is given by

$$j(r) = \frac{I}{4\pi r^2} \mathbf{u}_r. \tag{9}$$

The current gradient is then

$$\frac{di}{dr} = \frac{IA}{2\pi r^3},$$ (10)

and the threshold becomes

$$I_0 = \frac{3}{2} \frac{V_T}{\rho\lambda^2} \left(\frac{4}{3}\pi a^3\right),$$ (11)

where the electrode volume has been put in parentheses.

3. COMPARISON OF SPHERE AND CYLINDER

It is interesting to compare the thresholds of spherical and cylindrical electrodes. The above equations indicate that the thresholds continually become smaller with smaller electrodes; but as a practical matter, as will be shown later, electrode polarization (which has been neglected in this derivation) sets a lower limit on the size of the electrode that can be used. Thus a useful comparison is the ratio of the thresholds for the same surface area. The ratio so computed is also the ratio of current densities at the electrode surfaces for threshold stimulation. If this is done, the result is

$$\frac{\text{current density (sphere)}}{\text{current density (cylinder)}} = \frac{r_{\text{sphere}}}{2r_{\text{cylinder}}},$$ (12)

where the current densities are measured at threshold. Thus for the same radius at threshold a sphere has one-half the current density of a cylinder. Since the areas are to be the same for the two types of electrode, then $r^2_{\text{sphere}} = \frac{1}{2} l r_{\text{cylinder}}$, and the ratio of the currents at threshold is

$$\frac{I_{0\,\text{sphere}}}{I_{0\,\text{cylinder}}} = 0.35 \left(\frac{l}{r_{\text{cylinder}}}\right)^{\frac{1}{2}}.$$ (13)

The situation of (13) represents a case that may be tested experimentally. In many practical cases it can be seen that a sphere is more efficient than a cylinder; for example, consider the case of a cylindrical electrode whose length is twice its radius, so $l = 2r_{\text{cylinder}}$. The sphere of the same area then has a radius equal to the radius of the cylinder, but the threshold current for the sphere is one-half that of the cylinder. The sphere is actually somewhat smaller in overall size and has one-half the polarization of the cylinder [since it has one-half of the current density, as shown by (12)]. Most current pacemaker electrodes are basically cylinders, since the coiled spring now used so widely is, for electrical purposes, a cylinder. A spherical electrode would have superior performance, from the standpoint of both thresholds and polarization.

4. SURFACE ELECTRODES

A mathematical treatment of the thresholds of cardiac stimulation of surface electrodes is presented in this section. A result of the derivation is a proof that there is an optimum size for a surface electrode, a result confirmed experimentally.

A fundamental equation used, as in the previous development, is

$$(v - V) = \lambda^2 \frac{d^2v}{dx^2}. \tag{14}$$

Following the previous development, we replace d^2v/dx^2 (the derivative in the cell) by d^2V/dx^2 (the derivative in the medium external to the cell) because the perturbation of the field caused by the cell is small. Thus only the field produced by the electrodes and the surrounding tissue need by computed. The model used for calculating the fields is as follows: A perfectly conducting electrode is assumed to extend from $-c$ to $+c$ along the x-axis and to have a potential v_0 applied to it. The upper half-plane is a resistive tissue medium. The remainder of the x-axis is at zero potential. This implies that the surface of the heart, except for the electrode, is an equipotential surface. The strip is assumed to be infinitely long in the z-direction. This derivation basically represents the field for a long, thin electrode. It is desired to calculate the potential and the fields in the upper half-plane. Note that in the previous sections the electrode was not only at a uniform potential but had a constant current density. In the present case the current density is no longer constant. The electric potential for the assumed geometry is given by [9]

$$V(x,y) = \frac{1}{\pi} V_0 \left(\tan^{-1} \frac{c - x}{y} + \tan^{-1} \frac{c + x}{y} \right). \tag{15}$$

The electric field is computed by taking the gradient of the potential:

$$\mathbf{E} = \nabla V(x,y). \tag{16}$$

The result of this operation is

$$E = \frac{V_0}{\pi} \left\{ i y \left[\frac{1}{y^2 + (c+x)^2} - \frac{1}{y^2 + (c-x)^2} \right] \right.$$

$$\left. - j \left[\frac{c-x}{y^2 + (c-x)} + \frac{c+x}{y^2 + (c+x)} \right] \right\}, \quad (17)$$

where **i** and **j** are unit vectors in the x- and y-directions, respectively.

The formula for electric field exhibits the rate of change of potential both with x and y. Examination of these expressions shows that the voltage change between the cell core and the medium is a maximum if the cell lies along the x-axis. Assuming the cell lies along the x-axis,

$$\frac{d^2V}{dx^2} = -\frac{y^2 + (c-x)^2 + 2(c-x)^2}{[y^2 + (c-x)^2]^2}$$

$$+ \frac{y^2 + (c+x)^2 - 2(c+x)^2}{[y^2 + (c+x)^2]^2}. \quad (18)$$

It can be shown that this reaches its maximum for $x = \pm c$ (the edges of the electrode). At this point the value is

$$\frac{d^2V}{dx^2} = \frac{4cy}{(y^2 + 4c^2)^2}, \quad (19)$$

and the threshold is (where V_T is the threshold value of $v - V$, the transmembrane potential)

$$V_T = \frac{V_0 \lambda^2}{\pi} \frac{4cy}{(y^2 + 4c^2)^2} = (v - V)_{\text{th}}. \quad (20)$$

The differential is the same at $+c$ and $-c$ except for a change in sign, so the transmembrane potential will have the proper polarity at only one edge of the electrode. This equation has a maximum value for

$$c = \frac{y}{2\sqrt{3}}. \quad (21)$$

This may be interpreted in the following manner: If excitable cells were in contact (or very near) the electrode (corresponding to $y = 0$), then making the electrode very small would lower the electrode threshold (V_0) for a given cell threshold. This would be in agreement with the intuitive notion that increasing the current density would lower the threshold. However, as is well known, the epicardium is electrically insensitive; the closest sensitive cells are in the myocardium corresponding to a minimum value of *y.* When a surface electrode is used as an epicardial electrode, *y* has a minimum value equal to the distance between the surface of the epicardium and the nearest sensitive cells. There is thus an optimum electrode size.

From symmetry similar considerations apply to circular electrodes. For the strip electrode any plane perpendicular to the *z*-axis can be used as an *x-y* plane, whereas for the circular case any plane containing the *z*-axis can be used as an *x-y* plane.

This optimum cannot be verified experimentally for the endocardial electrode because the electrode cannot be repositioned accurately in the same place. However, the optimum has been shown to exist for surface electrodes [5].

As scar tissue forms *y* gradually increases. Thus the size of the electrode cannot be completely optimized in advance.

5. STRENGTH-DURATION CURVES

If the effects of membrane capacitance are included, then the characteristics of strength-duration curves may be computed and compared with experiments. The calculated curves quantitatively predict the shape of the curves and many parameters of interest, including the pulse width that gives minimum pacing energy and the effects of finite rise time on the pulses. The effects of various waveforms may also be computed, but this is not done here.

Levine [3] has performed a similar analysis based on a polynomial approximation to measured strength-duration curves. By contrast, the development here is based completely on theory and is related to the anatomical structure of the cell and its membrane.

First, it is shown that a cell may be approximately represented by a parallel *RC* circuit, as in Figure 5.3. If the cell is to be represented by this

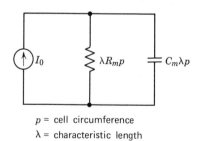

p = cell circumference
λ = characteristic length

Figure 5.3 Modified equivalent circuit of a cell used for deriving strength-duration curves.

simple lumped equivalent, then the outside of the cell is represented by the potential at a single external point, and the inside of the cell is represented by a single internal point, corresponding to the two nodes of the network. The cell exterior is an almost isopotential surface because of the high conductivity of the extracellular medium, and therefore the point selected is immaterial. This external potential changes, of course, when the stimulating pulse is applied. If the cell is initially depolarized, then its entire core is also all at the same potential. When a stimulating pulse is applied the potential in the external medium changes almost instantaneously (because the medium is resistive), but the core potential lags because of the membrane capacitance. Thus, initially the entire core is also at the same potential. The entire outside of the cell is, for all practical purposes, clamped at a fixed potential, and the potential of the core rises uniformly (except possibly near the ends) to meet it. It is assumed that this condition exists along at least one characteristic length (λ) of the cell.

It can then be shown [8] that because of the clamped external voltage the current entering the cell, I_0, and the transmembrane potential V_0 are related by (22) if capacitance is neglected:

$$\frac{V_0}{I_0} = \frac{R_m/\lambda}{p \tanh L/\lambda}, \tag{22}$$

where p is the cell circumference and the other terms have been previously defined. If $L \gg \lambda$, (22) reduces to

$$\frac{V_0}{I_0} = \frac{R_m}{\lambda p}. \tag{23}$$

If instead of the membrane resistance R_m we use the impedance per unit length, Z_m, which is given by

$$\frac{1}{Z_m} = \frac{1}{R_m} + sC_m, \tag{24}$$

where s is the Laplace operator and C_m is the membrane capacitance per square centimeter, we then have the operational relationship

$$\frac{V_0(s)}{I_0(s)} = \frac{1}{Z_m \lambda p}. \tag{25}$$

This represents the parallel combination of resistance and capacitance of the characteristic length of the membrane. The transfer function is that of the parallel RC circuit shown in Figure 5.3. Since these relations apply to a length λ of the cell, it can be seen that the assumptions concerning uniformity of potential need apply only to a region of this length, as was stated previously. It turns out that to reproduce the strength-duration curve the only parameter that must be known is the time constant of the cell. Hoffman and Cranefield [1] reported that this is about 2 msec for Purkinje fibers. This number, plus the rheobase thresholds of the previous section, permits derivation of the strength-duration curves.

As stated previously the electrodes set up an electric field in the intercellular medium, which produces a current across the cell membranes and depolarizes them. This process is represented as a current generator driving the RC combination of the cell. The exact magnitude of this current (which is the current entering the cell) is not important, because it turns out that the previous results concerning rheobase thresholds are all that is needed to determine the magnitudes of any effects. If the driving source is a rectangular pulse, the current pulse in the intercellular medium is rectangular also, since the medium is basically resistive. Thus the perturbing effects of the cell capacitance are neglected in determining the field at the cell. The transmembrane potential gradually builds up in response to the applied field; if the field is applied long enough, the transmembrane potential reaches threshold, and the cell depolarizes. A strength-duration curve is the relationship between the magnitude of the intensity of the threshold stimulus and its duration when they are both at a level that is sufficient to make the cell fire. The cell parameters change after the cell has depolarized, but they remain constant until that time.

If a step of current is applied to the circuit of Figure 5.3, then the voltage V across the membrane is related to the amplitude of the driving current step, I_0, by the relation

$$V = I_0 R_m (1 - e^{-d/T}), \tag{26}$$

where T is the time constant of the combination. At threshold $V = V_{th}$ and $t = d$, the pulse width. Thus for a single cell we have

$$I_0 = \frac{V_{th}}{R(1 - e^{-d/T})}. \tag{27}$$

Note that this is the current entering the cell: it is *not* the current supplied by the electrode. However, since the tissue is basically resistive (neglecting polarization effects), this current is proportional to the current from the electrode. If I_{el} is the current supplied by the electrode and I_R is the rheobase current computed in the previous section, then we can say that, since I_{el} is proportional to I_0,

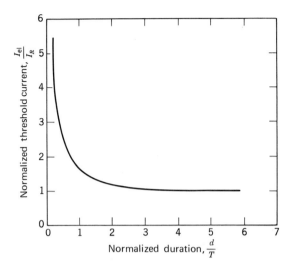

Figure 5.4 Theoretical current strength duration curve. Vertical axis is the ratio of the current supplied to rheobase current, whereas the horizontal axis is the ratio of the pulse width to cell time constant.

$$I_{el} = \frac{I_R}{(1 - e^{-d/T})}. \qquad (28)$$

This relationship is plotted in Figure 5.4. The time scale in this figure is d/T, or stimulus duration divided by the cell time constant. This method of normalization has been used to simplify comparison of the experimental data with the theory. In addition, such a normalization in effect makes the figure a "universal curve," which can be used for cells with different time constants.

The energy required may also be computed. If the pacemaker is a current generator, then I_{el} is a constant. If R_0 is the resistance of the tissue as seen by the electrode, then the energy per pulse U is given by

$$U = I_{el}{}^2 \, R_0 = \frac{dI_R{}^2 R_0}{(1 - e^{-d/T})^2}. \qquad (29)$$

This relationship is plotted in Figure 5.5. It has a minimum at about $1.4T$. Using the figure of 2.8 msec for T quoted by Hoffman and Cranefield, we find that the optimum pulse width is about 1.6 msec. Most pacemakers in use today have pulse widths between 1 and 3 msec, and thus are very close

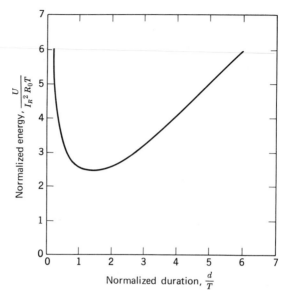

Figure 5.5   Theoretical energy strength duration curve; normalization used is same as Figure 5.4.

to optimum. The pulse widths in actual use have been determined from several years of experience, and thus it would be quite surprising if they were not near the optimum value. Note that the minimum is quite broad, so that the actual width is not critical from this standpoint. This result agrees with a recent experimental study by Furman [4].

6.   EXPERIMENTAL VERIFICATION

The theoretical results presented here were compared with experimental data both qualitatively and quantitatively. The qualitative verification consists of showing that pacemaker thresholds do depend on the volume of the implanted electrode, and that the relationship between spherical and cylindrical electrodes is as shown. This was done with cylindrical myocardial electrodes such as those shown in Figure 5.6, in which a cylinder of metal is insulated at both ends with silicone rubber (to minimize end effects), and with electrodes that are basically spherical "blobs" of metal. A series of these were serially implanted in the heart of an experimental animal, and the thresholds were measured. It was important to measure all of the thresholds in one animal because of the known variations between animals, but this procedure limited the number of electrodes that could be measured at any one time. It was found to be impractical to make more than four measurements because of the small size of the dog's heart and the traumatic effect of the repeated wounds for the electrodes. Thus a basic problem with the experiments is that each curve has only a small number of points (three or four) through which a variety of curves can be drawn. The basic verification comes from the quantitative agreement of the theory and the experiments. Although it would be desirable to have more points, the experimental problems seem to preclude this. It was not practical to verify these results with endocardial electrodes because of the difficulty of insuring that each of the electrodes lay in the same place in the interior of the heart.

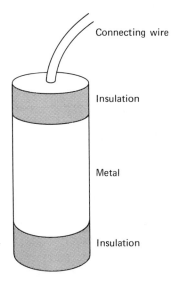

Figure 5.6 Sketch showing details of construction of experimental electrodes.

Exact quantitative verification is much more difficult because of the uncertainty of the magnitudes of the parameters in the various equations. Some of these parameters are known fairly well for cardiac cells, but others are almost completely unknown in the forms necessary. It is also necessary to have the data for dogs, since they were used as experimental subjects. Many of the measurements that have been made on cardiac cells and that might be applicable have given only the total resistance and capacitance of the cells on which they were measured, making it difficult to obtain the various parameters in normalized form. To obtain a rough check a set of numbers was compiled from various references, modifying some to make them consistent with each other and with various known parameters of the heart. These numbers, which at best can be considered to be only estimates, are presented in Table 1 and were used for the theoretical curves plotted in this section. In view of the known variation from animal to animal in thresholds and the approximate nature of these constants, the quantitative agreement of the theory with the experiments seems to be reasonably good. A more exact check must await more precise determination of the constants.

Tests were run on seven dogs. Figure 5.7 shows the results for one dog with cylindrical electrodes compared with the theoretical values as computed from the parameters of Table 1. The data were taken with a pulse width of 1 msec, so the theoretical curve has been modified by using the data of Figure 5.4 to get a rheobase threshold. The diameters of the electrodes varied from 2.05 to 3.8 mm, and the lengths varied from 8.0 to 12.6 mm. In spite of the fact that the electrode diameters are not always much greater than the space constant of the cells, the agreement is reasonably good, indicating that the assumption concerning the relative sizes of the electrode and the space constant may not be a necessary condition. In this particular case six electrodes were serially implanted in the dog within a period of 2 hours, so that we might expect the response of the dog to change during the period of the experiment. Other experiments were run with smaller number of electrodes, and these also conformed to the theoretical results.

A few experiments were made to determine whether a spherical electrode was superior to a cylindrical one. The major problem here was fabricating the spheres to reasonable tolerances and sizes. Also, the cylindrical electrodes were always long as compared to their radius, to minimize end effects. However, the cases measured showed that spherical electrodes had a lower threshold than the cylindrical ones for a given volume, although the data showed more scatter when compared with theory.

7.   CONCLUSIONS

The theoretical results presented here describe the variation of threshold currents with cardiac pacemaker electrodes. They generally agree with experimental results. It should be noted that from a completely experimental basis it is possible to fit a straight line to the threshold values if they are either plotted against the area of the electrode or if they are plotted against the implanted volume of the electrode. The significance of the results presented

TABLE 1.   Parameters Used to Compute Theoretical Curve
of Threshold Versus Volume

Threshold voltage of cell, V_{th}	50 mV
Characteristic length of cell, λ	2 mm
Resistivity of cell core, ρ_c	150 ohm-cm

Note: $I_{th} = \dfrac{V_{th}}{\rho_c \lambda^2} (2\pi l a^2)$ for cylindrical electrodes.

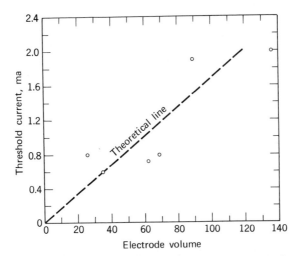

Stimulation threshold versus Electrode volume, mm³

Figure 5.7 Comparison of theoretical and experimental results for a dog.

here is that the theory permits us to calculate the magnitudes of the threshold currents and not to rely entirely on the experimental data. The theory also predicts differences in thresholds for electrodes with different shapes. This can also be verified experimentally and cannot be explained by the notion that the threshold depends on surface area alone. Qualitatively, however, this theory verifies the well-known fact that smaller electrodes have lower thresholds of stimulation.

When the electrode becomes smaller its threshold decreases; however, the polarization voltages increase, and thus the pacing energy increases. Thus there is an optimum size electrode from the standpoint of pacemaker energy. This optimum size depends on whether the threshold varies with the radius squared or the radius cubed of the electrode.

REFERENCES

[1] Hoffman, B., and C. Cranefield, *Electrophysiology of the Heart*, McGraw-Hill, New York, 1960.
[2] Mansfield, P., and A. Cole, "Design and Analysis of Myocardial Electrodes," *Proc. 16th Ann. Conf. Med. in Eng. and Biol.*, 1963.

[3] Levine, N., "Electrochemical Behavior of Metals as Stimulus Electrodes," *J. Biol. Med. Mat'l, Res.,* 1:1, March 1967.

[4] Furman, S., A. Denize, D. Escher, and J. Schwebel, "Energy Consumption for Cardiac Stimulation as a Function of Pulse Duration," *J. Surg. Res.,* 6:10, October 1966.

[5] Lewin, G., G. H. Myers, V. Parsonnet, and I. R. Zucker, "A Non-Polarizing Electrode for Physiological Stimulation," *Trans. ASA,* 10, XIII, 1967.

[6] Lale, P. G., "Muscular Contraction by Implanted Stimulators," *Med. Biol. Eng.,* 4:4, July 1966.

[7] Katz, B., *Nerve, Muscle, and Synapse,* McGraw-Hill, New York, 1960.

[8] Loewenstein, W., "Permeability of Membrane Junctions," *Ann. N. Y. Acad. Sci.,* 137 (Art. 2) (1966).

[9] Hildebrand, F., *Advanced Calculus for Engineers,* Prentice-Hall, Englewood Cliffs, N. J., 1949.

CHAPTER SIX

Pacemaker Electrodes

The pacemaker electrodes are at the interface between the electronics of the pacemaker and the heart, and thus they play a key role in pacemaker operation. This interface is a sensitive area in which many problems may arise with the electrodes, the leads joining the electrodes to the pacemaker itself, or in the tissues. Many of the phenomena do not occur until a long time has elapsed and as a result are still poorly understood.

Two types of problems arise with the electrodes and the leads: those that are purely mechanical and those that might be termed *electrobiological*. The mechanical problems include avoidance of metal fatigue of leads, including proper implantation procedures, and designing leak-proof joints to the package containing the electronics portion of the pacemaker. The solutions to some of these can be obtained by conventional engineering forms of analysis. The electrobiological problems include a gradual rise in stimulation thresholds, scar tissue formation around the electrode surfaces, corrosion (since these are often related to biological and biochemical reactions), and proper stimulating waveforms. There is a considerable lack of information in the last area.

1. TYPES OF ELECTRODE

The first pacemakers used electrodes external to the body cavities, attached to the surface of the thorax [1]. However, so high a voltage was required for this method (over 100 volts) and the discomfort to the patient from the electric shock and twitching of the muscles of the chest wall was so great that it was soon abandoned except for emergency purposes. The next step employed external circuitry, and wires were led to the heart through the skin. However, the points where the wires passed through the skin became portals for infection, and therefore this method was set aside except for certain situations that are discussed later.

Implantable pacemakers, the devices of choice for long-term pacing, have two wires running from them to the myocardium. Alternatively a catheter is passed through a vein into the interior of the right ventricle (endocardial pacing). Thus the fundamental difference between these two methods is that in one case the stimulation is directly in the muscle bundle of the heart, and in the other it is on the interior surface of the ventricles. Either of these lead systems may be used with any of the types of pacemakers that transmit their energy into the body by radio means, but the pacemaker in this case must incorporate a receiving coil in its circuit. At this time research is being conducted on pacemakers that can be sutured directly onto the heart. Such a procedure will minimize some of the mechanical problems such as fatigue but will not reduce the electrobiological ones, and it may produce some problems of its own.

Catheter electrodes, to be considered first, may be either bipolar (i.e., have two electrodes at the catheter tip) or monopolar (only one electrode at the catheter tip). An indifferent, or reference, electrode (similar to a ground in ordinary circuits) somewhere in the body is necessary if monopolar electrodes are used. Figure 6.1 shows monopolar, bipolar, and tripolar electrodes. In a bipolar catheter the two electrodes are usually 1 cm apart. The tripolar electrode (three electrodes on the catheter surface) is usually used with the two

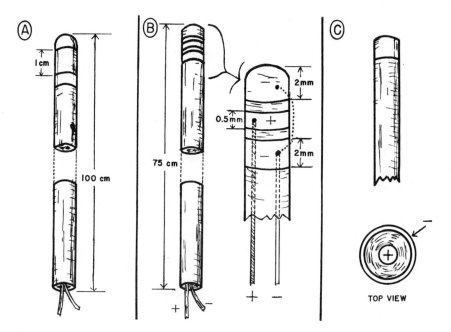

Figure 6.1   Schematic drawing of types of Electrodes. A–bipolar, B–tripolar, C–coaxial.

end electrodes joined. The coaxial electrode has one of its electrodes in the flat end of the catheter. Other bipolar electrodes have been used with the poles 3 to 4 cm apart or with a long leading tip advanced ahead of the bipole.

A monopolar electrode, of course, has just one electrode surface at the catheter tip. In general the bipolar and monopolar catheters have proved themselves to be most effective in practice. The other types of electrodes were fabricated in an attempt to produce greater current densities in the responsive tissue in the heart adjacent to the electrodes. It was felt that the tripolar electrode might be less sensitive to placement in the heart, since the current flow is in two directions from the center band. If the coaxial catheter is placed with its tip directly against the heart wall, then the current flow all passes through the tissue. In practice it has been found that any advantage these electrode forms had were marginal or nonexistent.

Catheter electrodes were originally used exclusively with external pacemakers in emergency procedures. Their great advantage is that insertion into the heart does not require a thoracotomy, and they can be inserted under a local anesthetic. Thus, if a patient is admitted to the hospital with heart block and in a weakened condition, as is usually the case, a catheter can be inserted transvenously and connected to an external pacemaker. Pacing can be continued for a period of days or months (or even years) until the patient has recovered sufficiently to allow implantation of a pacemaker with myocardial leads. The success of such transvenous pacing has been so great that special pacemakers and catheters were developed that could be implanted. Often the temporary catheter could be used for the permanent device. The implanted pacemaker could also be placed under the skin rather than in the chest itself, thereby considerably reducing the magnitude of the surgical procedure required.

The theory of electrode stimulation presented in Chapter 5 should apply to internal bipolar electrodes. The geometry is much more complex, however, since the electrode tips are constantly bathed in a conducting fluid (blood), and it would seem that there would be a tendency for them to be shorted out. That this does not happen is shown by the fact that internal electrodes usually require less energy to stimulate the heart than do external ones. It seems likely that the electrodes themselves must touch the surface of the heart to achieve maximum stimulation (or lowest threshold), although there have been some reports of stimulation without contact. At any rate, it is almost impossible to place the electrodes in the ventricle without having them touch the heart surface at one time or another. If the motion of the fluid is neglected, then the electric field produced by these electrodes can be computed by the principles of electrostatics. Such a map is indicated in Figure 6.2 for

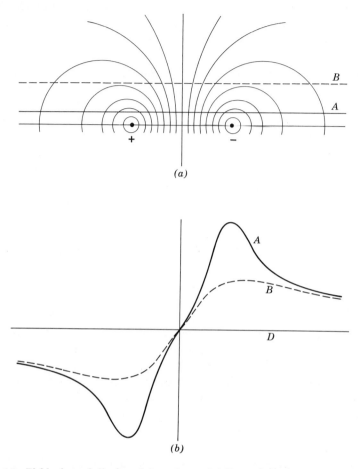

Figure 6.2 Field plots of dipoles: (*a*) equipotential lines of dipole used to represent bipolar catheter; (*b*) electric field along lines *A* and *B* of (*a*).

a bipolar electrode. For a monopolar electrode, the field lines would probably be more nearly radial.

The actual stimulation seems to be caused by current entering responsive tissue [2]. This is suggested by the fact that as scar tissue builds up over the electrode ends, forming an insulating coating (as shown in the insert of Figure 6.6*a*), the threshold for stimulation rises, although the electrical resistance at the electrode end remains approximately constant. This suggests that the electrode is being removed from viable tissue, with the result that the current density at this viable tissue is diminished. The fact that thresholds also do not rise as high with monopolar as with bipolar electrodes tends to support this theory.

Although many pacemakers today use catheter electrodes, most still have the more conventional myocardial electrodes that are sewn into the muscle of the ventricles. These wires are usually made from platinum-iridium or stainless-steel wire wound in a spiral and insulated with silicone rubber, polyethylene, or Teflon. Others are of stranded stainless steel plated with gold or platinum. In both the catheter and direct myocardial electrodes fatigue is a considerable problem because the leads flex with each heartbeat. In a year the heart beats more than 40 million times. Fatigue problems are more severe with external electrodes. Thus an electrode material must have good fatigue resistance, low electrical resistance, and be nonreactive in the body.

There are not many materials that meet these requirements, and the two most successful have been platinum-iridium and some alloys, particularly Elgiloy. In general stainless steels have shown superior fatigue resistance, but unfortunately corrosion occurs at a stainless-steel anode. Therefore, if steel is used, it must be employed as the cathode, which is connected to the heart; a remote disk acting as an indifferent electrode is used as the anode. The disk can be made large enough to make corrosion negligible.

The fact that corrosion takes place is interesting, because, as will be discussed later, the pulse generators are coupled to the heart through a capacitor, so that no direct current can flow. Thus the terms "anode" and "cathode" do not really apply to these electrodes in the conventional sense but can only be applied on a "per pulse" basis. In some pacemakers a slight negative potential is applied to the cathode to inhibit corrosion. Some sort of nonlinear rectification may take place at the junction between the heart and the electrodes.

One of the first pacemaker electrodes to be used were employed by Hunter and Roth in 1959. The electrodes were two stainless-steel pins 0.5 cm long that projected from the bottom of a small, flat, rectangular piece of silicone rubber. The lead wire was made of Teflon-coated multistrand stainless steel that was insulated by an outer sleeve of silicone-rubber tubing. With this electrode a large number of failures occurred from fatigue; one of the causes was the stress concentration caused by the welding together of two different metals. Tests also showed that accommodation to slight elongation would also be desirable. As a result most pacemakers in use today (although not all) use what has come to be known as the Chardack electrode, illustrated in Figures 6.3 and 6.4. As originally built by Chardack [3], the electrode material was platinum-iridium, but the same design has been used with stainless steel. Both loose and tight coils have been employed. In the electrodes used by Chardack the conducting element is a helical coil of platinum-iridium

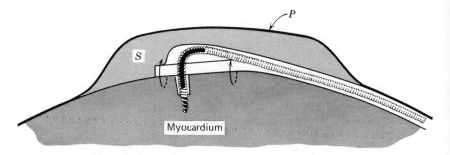

Figure 6.3   Method of fixation of electrodes on ventricular myocardium. (Courtesy of W. Chardack.)

alloy 0.010 in. in diameter. The diameter of the coil itself is 0.044 in., and it extends in one piece from the pacemaker terminal to the electrode plate where it turns and terminates as the electrode pin, which is a section of the coil itself. The use of a single continuous structure eliminates all junctions of dissimilar metals and prevents corrosion from galvanic action as well as the stress concentrations created by such joints. Resistance to fatigue caused by bending is greatly increased by use of the coiled-spring configuration.

The details of the construction of the electrode plate are shown in Figure 6.4. At the point where the coil makes the turn it is stabilized by a solid platinum-iridium wire core. Two-thirds of the portion of the coil that projects as the electrode is insulated by a silicone-rubber sleeve, which limits the electrode area in order to produce a high current density at the electrode tip. The last three turns of the coil are opened slightly to permit fibrous tissue

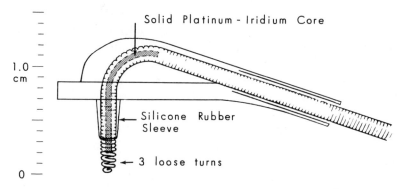

Figure 6.4   Detail of electrode tips of myocardial electrode. (Courtesy of W. Chardack.)

to grow between the spirals and thus hold the tip in place. The silicone-rubber electrode support has four predrilled holes that are used for suturing it to the myocardium.

The methods used for inserting and fixing the electrode to the myocardium are shown in Figure 6.3. A stab wound is made into the myocardium at the insertion point; this wound must be placed accurately with respect to the suture holes so that there will be no twist on the electrode tip when the silicone-rubber disk that supports the electrodes is anchored with the sutures. The electrode is pushed into the stab wound and is held in place while the sutures are tied down. It is essential to avoid bending or twisting the electrode pin during this process, because deformation may lead to the creation of a point of weakness in a critical area and may eventually lead to a fatigue failure. Sufficient length of electrode leads must be left to form a strain-relieving loop to prevent fatigue failure. Sharp corners must be avoided.

It is interesting to note that most of these insertion problems do not have to be considered in the case of the catheter electrodes, simply because there is little that can be done about them. The catheter follows the curve of the vein through which it is inserted, and it is therefore impossible to leave strain-relief loops or to avoid corners that may be present in the veins themselves. Where the catheter electrode traverses the atrium, however, a strain-relieving loop is desirable; the size of this loop is determined by the judgment of the surgeon based upon the degree of electrode movement seen on the fluoroscope, heart size, and the relationship of the position of the catheter to the tricuspid value ring where considerable distortion of the catheter frequently is encountered. In general the stresses on catheter electrodes seem to be somewhat smaller than those on myocardial electrodes because the right ventricle containing the catheter moves somewhat less forcefully than the left, in which direct wires are usually placed.

2. STIMULATION PHENOMENA

A basic theory of pacemaker stimulation was presented in the preceding chapter. There are several additional phenomena that affect the stimulation process in any practical case:

1. Electrode polarization effects occur at the interface between the metal and the electrolyte of the body fluids, and absorb a large amount of energy.

2. Scar tissue that eventually forms about the electrode implantation sites affects the amount of energy and charge required.

3. The location of responsive cells varies with respect to the electrodes.

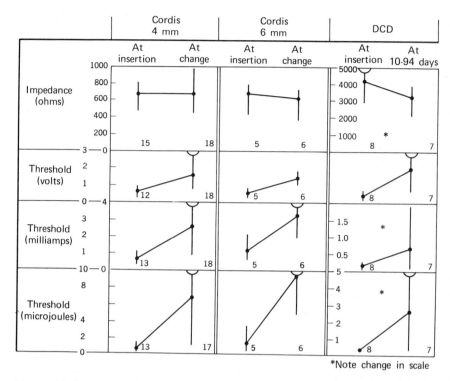

Figure 6.5 Data taken by the authors showing variations in different threshold parameters for different electrodes from insertion to time of pacemaker change. See text for discussion.

To put these matters in the proper perspective, it may be recalled from the section on the physiology of stimulation that the action potential is on the order of 0.1 volt. Approximately 0.05 volt is sufficient to depolarize a cardiac cell.

The threshold of implanted electrodes reaches a peak in about 10 days and then gradually falls to a lower plateau where it tends to remain thereafter (unless some abnormal reaction occurs that will alter the amount of scar tissue). Figure 6.5 presents some data taken by the authors that indicate how various parameters relating to thresholds change between implantation and removal of pacemakers. The data are given for two different size Cordis catheter electrodes, and the DCD electrode described in more detail later in this chapter. Changes in threshold, impedance, current, voltage, and energy are given. The voltage threshold is measured with a voltage source, whereas the current threshold is measured with a current source. The small numbers in each box indicate the number of cases used in arriving at the values given, which in all cases show the means and range (shown by the vertical line through the point). Note that not all scales start at zero. The time interval between the two points varies with the pacemaker but is usually on the order of several years. The first point is taken while the patient is still in the hospital, before the initial increase has occurred. (The initial increase can be measured while the patient is in the hospital by not implanting the pacemaker until the increase has occurred.) As might be expected, small electrodes have lower thresholds than large ones, and the change in threshold is relatively unaffected by the electrode size. Note, however, that the impedance changes are in general negligible and appear to be uncorrelated with the threshold changes.

The increase in threshold may be responsible for lack of stimulation in some cases. The stimulation threshold rises, whereas the voltage available gradually falls as the batteries begin to age. Eventually, these two characteristics cross, resulting in the pacemaker's being unable to pace the heart.

The rise in threshold is generally accompanied by and is probably due to the growth of scar tissue [2] about the electrode ends. The thickness of the scar (fibrous) tissue determines the amount of rise in threshold. The reasons for this can be explained on the basis of the theory presented in the preceding chapter. Immediately after implantation active cells are in close proximity to the electrodes. The effective electrode size therefore corresponds to its actual physical size. As the fibrous tissue grows this layer of nonresponsive tissue insulates the electrode from the nearest responsive tissue. Effectively, the outer surface of the scar tissue (which is a conductor, as are most body tissues) becomes the electrode. However, the electrode size is now much greater, and so the current density and electric field in the tissue are lowered because the total amount of current available from the pacemaker is basically constant. Measurements made by the authors indicate that the impedance at the electrode tips is almost independent of stimulation threshold. This effect is illustrated schematically in Figure 6.6, which shows the fibrous tissue forming the nonresponsive barrier and thus moving the effective electrode out further from the metallic electrode. The phenomenon is clearly similar to that which takes place with the catheter electrodes described previously.

It was originally thought that the rise in threshold was due to an increase in the electrical impedance of the tissues with time. Thus, if the pacemaker were a constant voltage source, which is true of some existing pacemakers, an increasing voltage would be required to provide the same stimulating current, because of the increased impedance. As a result of this the circuits of many pacemakers were changed to high-impedance sources (current sources). Figure 6.5 shows that the impedance rise, although present, is not very large (on the order of 20 percent) and that the threshold increases even with a

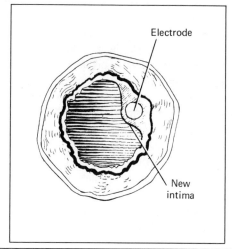

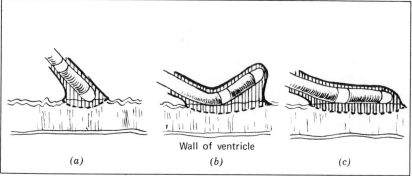

Figure 6.6   Sketch of growth of scar tissue about electrodes, believed to be the cause of threshold increase.

constant-current stimulator. Thus the fibrous tissue theory presented here seems to be the most likely explanation at this time.

From the previous discussion it can be seen that two problems must be solved if more efficient pacing methods are to be designed:

1. A method must be found to minimize scar tissue growth.

2. Methods must be found for stimulating with lower voltages and currents that more nearly approach the thresholds of single cells.

It is a fact that almost any foreign body in the tissues causes fibrous tissue to form. This effect, known as the foreign body reaction, is ubiquitous, appearing not only with artificial substances but also with transplants and with wounds. Even completely inert materials cause scar tissue to form, so the problem of pacemaker electrodes is just a small part of the overall problem. Electrical stimulation itself may be traumatic to the tissues and encourage a fibrous-tissue reaction. When metal electrodes are used some of the metal goes into solution at the electrode ends because of the high current densities involved, which may also aggravate the effect. This passing of ions into solution occurs even with platinum, which is one of the most inert substances known. It has been proposed that the cause of the fibrous tissue is impurities that happen to be at the electrode tip at implantation and irritate the healthy tissue. These impurities may include powder from the surgeon's gloves and minute particles of sterile dirt that interrupt the smoothness of the surfaces. Such minute impurities are extremely difficult to eliminate because of the difficulty of scouring the delicate leads, which might damage them and make them unfit for implantation. Powder is used to keep surgical gloves from sticking when they are put on, and as a result is present almost everywhere in the operating room. A solution to this problem is to supply pacemakers with leads that have been thoroughly cleaned at the factory and have been presterilized. The Adcole leads come attached to gauze pads to provide a "handle" for the surgeon so that it becomes unnecessary to touch the electrodes themselves. One objection to this practice, even assuming its correctness, is that these measures may be difficult to accomplish in the average operating room. If it is true that even touching the electrode tips will cause scar tissue to form, we can easily envision cases in which they will become inadvertently "contaminated" with powder merely by exposing them to the air.

Even if all fibrous reaction could be prevented, however, it would probably still remain a fact that the stimulation thresholds would be considerably greater than would be predicted by the electrophysical phenomena measured in the cell. The explanation for this lies in polarization at the electrodes and by size limitations on electrodes. Polarization is produced largely by reaction products at the electrodes. This effect was a limiting one in early chemical batteries, in which the principal reaction product that limited the voltage was hydrogen. It was eliminated in batteries by the use of substances called depolarizers, but no feasible way has been found to use such a technique with stimulating electrodes, where the electrolyte is the blood and body tissues.

Although the chemistry and physics of the polarization phenomena are a complete subject in themselves and therefore cannot be covered in detail here, the effect is of such importance in pacemakers and other physiological stimulators that a brief review of the pertinent facts is included. The subject is actually important not only for stimulators but also for electrodes used for making electrical measurements in the body, such as the microelectrodes previously described that were used for measuring cellular transmembrane potentials. In these cases the back emf produced by polarization affects any static (non-time-varying) voltages that may be measured.

As was noted in a previous chapter, differences in charge densities between the two sides of an interface produce a potential difference across that interface. If two liquids are in apposition, in general a membrane between them is required to prevent diffusion of the two liquids and eventual disappearance of the potential. In the case of a metal in an electrolyte, however, a natural boundary exists. Charge densities and mobilities are different in the two media, and thus a potential barrier forms at the interface and affects the flow of current. The effect is similar to that which is responsible for the barrier at a transistor junction. The barrier that forms across the metal-electrolyte interface is known as the *double layer* and acts in a manner similar to a large leaky capacitor (capacitances on the order of 50 μf have been measured for typical electrodes). The capacitance, however, is nonlinear. Any static potentials that exist because of polarization are usually quite small (on the order of millivolts) and are not of importance in pacemaker phenomena, since any constant voltage at the electrodes does not affect the operation of the pacemaker because of the coupling capacitor that prevents direct currents from flowing between the pacemaker and the tissues. The capacitor, however, can become charged from the pacemaker output and affect the waveforms of the current and voltage. In addition, since polarization is caused by electrochemical effects, polarization will cause corrosion at sufficiently high current densities. Thus the size of electrodes cannot be indefinitely decreased because then the current densities approach values sufficiently high to cause them to disintegrate. Actually, several effects take place at the interface at different levels of current density. At low current densities the principal cause of polarization is the charge-concentration gradients that have just been discussed. After a certain threshold in current density is reached other effects begin to operate, and corrosion appears, even with alternating currents. In pacemaker electrodes the current density is sufficiently high so that, if bipolar electrodes are used, corrosion can occur at the anode with many metals, even though the pacemaker output is alternating current (through a capacitor) coupled to the tissue, and no direct current can flow. In the case of monopolar electrode stimulation the anode has a large area, the current density is low, and there is no or little corrosion. In general corrosion does not occur at cathodes. It is fortunate that this is the case, because tissue seems to be slightly more responsive to negative stimulating pulses than to positive stimulating pulses.

Excellent studies of the effects of electrode polarization and its effects on pacemakers are those of Greatbatch and of Weinman and Mahler [3, 4]. Greatbatch first verified that he could reproduce pacemaker voltage and current waveforms in normal saline solution if approximately 200 ohms were

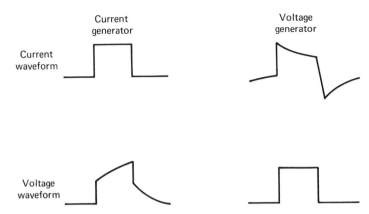

Figure 6.7 Effects of electrode polarization on pacemaker waveforms.

added in series with the leads (the actual value of resistance would be different for different tissue specimens). The voltage and current waveforms actually observed are shown in Figure 6.7, which distinguishes between voltage and current sources for the driving generators. If a square wave of current is used it is found that the voltage first jumps to an initial value and then increases slowly with an approximately exponential waveform to some asymptote. When the current waveform drops off the voltage waveform drops abruptly by an amount equal to its initial rise and then again decays exponentially. If a voltage source is used, the initial current is a high spike whose amplitude depends on the rise time of the applied voltage waveform. It can be seen that responses such as those indicated will be caused by an equivalent load of the type indicated in Figure 6.8, consisting of a resistance in parallel with a series resistor and capacitor. The value of the capacitor, as noted previously, is on the order of 5 to 25 μf [3]. The two resistances are necessary to explain the time constants measured with voltage and current sources. (Note that the effect of a shunt resistor with a current source differs from that with a voltage source.) There is some evidence to indicate that a very large capacitance should be in series with the first resistor also and that a true "lumped circuit" representation of the polarization effects would involve a ladder of resistors and capacitors. The values of the elements in these circuits are current dependent, as shown by Schwan [5].

It is generally believed that the current through the first resistor in the equivalent circuit is responsible for the tissue stimulation. However, even this is not completely true because some polarization effects manifest themselves as ohmic resistance which cannot be accounted for by bulk effects in the conductor. It can be seen that if a current source is used to produce

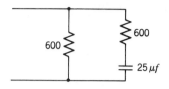

Figure 6.8 A typical equivalent circuit representing a pacemaker load. The actual nonlinear elements are here shown as fixed resistors and capacitors.

the driving pulse, the initial voltage rise just referred to consists of current through the two resistors in parallel. Because the resistor that is not in series with the capacitor is much smaller than the other one, most of the current goes through it.

Greatbatch's main experiment to show the effect of polarization in pacemakers was carried out in saline solution with the setup just described. He placed two pacemaker electrodes in the fluid and measured potentials near them with silver-silver chloride electrodes, which have very low polarization and are often used as standards (but unfortunately cannot be used as biological electrodes because they produce toxic reactions after about 20 min of use). He found that the potentials measured by the pickup electrodes in the fluid were on the order of a few tenths of a volt when the stimulating pulses were several volts. The pickup electrodes were approximately 1 mm away from the stimulating electrodes. Thus almost all of the voltage was dissipated at the electrode surface. If a current source was used, the stimulation was maintained at the desired value, but the polarization potential meant that more voltage was used to maintain the desired current.

Greatbatch [3] also measured the polarization potentials for several widely used pacemaker-electrode materials at typical pacemaker current densities and with pacemaker waveforms (see Figure 6.9). It can be seen that platinum is very good and that Elgiloy, which is widely used, has a much higher back voltage. As a matter of fact, it is not possible to use Elgiloy for bipolar electrodes, because the anode will corrode. Thus, if Elgiloy is used, it is necessary to provide a large-area indifferent electrode as an anode in order to keep the current density sufficiently low.

An electrode that overcomes many of the problems previously discussed is the differential-current-density (DCD) electrode developed at the Newark Beth Israel Hospital by the authors and Dr. Gerhard Lewin [6]. This electrode has a threshold of stimulation that is considerably lower than that of a conventional metal electrode. The energy required is about one-twentieth that of the usual pacemaker electrode. The current required goes down by about a factor of 10; and the voltage, by a factor of 2. The increase in threshold for chronic implantation is about the same as with metal electrodes.

The basic idea behind the differential-current-density electrode is to produce a low current density at the metal-electrolyte interface and a high cur-

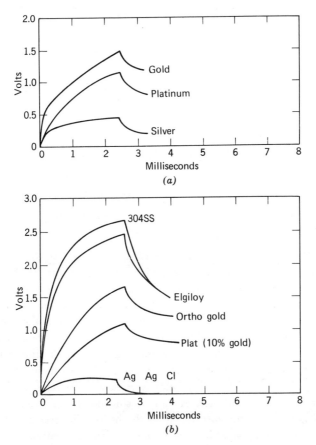

Figure 6.9 Voltages developed across various electrodes by three milliampere constant current pulse showing effects of polarization: (*a*) noble metal; (*b*) alloyed metal. (After Greatbatch.)

rent density at the tissue to be stimulated. The method for doing this is shown in Figure 6.10, which shows both a surface electrode (which can be used at the tip of a catheter) and a myocardial electrode. A cup is filled with normal saline solution or another biologically inert electrolyte and a large-area metal electrode (usually a piece of platinum with an area of 1 cm^2) is placed in it. A hole with a surface area of approximately 0.5 mm^2 is in contact with the tissue. In the case of the myocardial electrode the hole is at the end of a small projection that extends into the tissue. Since all of the current that leaves the metal disk must pass through the hole, it may be seen

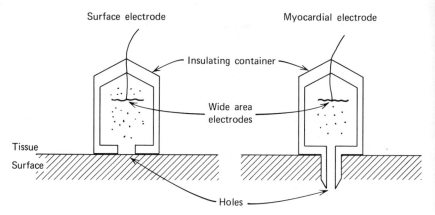

Figure 6.10 Sketch showing principles of operation of differential current density (DCD) electrode.

that it is a simple matter to have a high current density at the hole and a low current density at the metal. The saline solution is evidently soon replaced by body fluids, since these electrodes have been implanted chronically and continued to operate properly. It might appear that the hole could be made indefinitely small, and thus that the threshold could be decreased to the theoretical minimum. Both experimental evidence and the theoretical presentation of the planar electrode in the preceding chapter show that there is an optimum hole size and that thresholds start to increase once the hole becomes smaller than this critical size. A cuff of silicone rubber around the surface electrode is provided for suturing it to the heart. Catheter electrodes of this type are somewhat more difficult to insert than conventional ones because of the necessity of insuring that the hole is in contact with the responsive tissue. Once the catheter has been properly placed and left undisturbed for a few weeks, connective tissue grows around it and holds it in proper position.

3.   MECHANICAL PROBLEMS

There are three principal nonbiological problems associated with present leads: (a) corrosion, (b) fatigue, and (c) seals to the pacemaker assembly. The corrosion problem is closely related to the polarization phenomena previously discussed. The principal cause of corrosion is polarization if identical metals are used for cathode and anode. As discussed in the previous section, this problem can be solved completely if the cathode is used for stimulation and the anode has a large area. Noble-metal electrodes (such as platinum) can be used for either anodes or cathodes. However, some newer types of electrodes, which have been developed to achieve improved fatigue resistance, use dissimilar metals, and with these there is a danger that galvanic action will cause electrode corrosion. Because these newer types of electrodes are designed to solve the fatigue problem, their corrosion characteristics will be discussed under that heading.

The fatigue problem arises because of the enormous number of times the lead must flex; that is, at least once a second due to the heartbeat, not including its more complex three-dimensional oscillation, in addition to the motions caused by the diaphragm, and muscles of the chest and abdomen with which they make contact. At this time the most successful lead configuration for fatigue resistance has been the coiled spring, which has been fabricated from both platinum-iridium and from Elgiloy. If sufficient care is taken in the handling and insertion of this electrode, it seems fair to say that fatigue fracture will be rare. The manufacturers report lead breakages at less than 2.5 percent, and it is probable that some of these result from improper handling.

The spring must never be allowed to become kinked or bent. Any shock, such as comes from being dropped on the floor, is sufficient cause for not using the device, even if there is no apparent damage. Similarly, care must be taken during implantation to ensure that sharp bends are not created and that excess stress is not produced accidentally. Stress-relief loops in the length between the electronics and the heart should be included. However, there is some doubt concerning their effectiveness, because the leads eventually become trapped in a tissue sheath that prevents free movement of the loops. However, leaving a certain amount of shock relief accommodates initial movement of the pacemaker until the patient resumes normal activity after the operation, and presumably the leads will then assume "comfortable" curves and loops.

Several attempts have been made to develop a sturdier lead that will not require so much care in handling. One of the more interesting of these has been developed by the Brunswick Corporation for the Electrodyne pacemaker. The basic material is a yarn whose fiber is made from Elgiloy. Since the strands of the yarn are limp, we would expect that the stresses, and therefore the fatigue, would be very low, and this seems to be the case. The filament of Elgiloy is spun into a yarn and impregnated with silicone rubber under high pressure. The Elgiloy yarn is actually the strength-bearing core of the pacemaker. The conductor of the electrical current is a platinum wire, which is wound spirally around the silicone-impregnated core. The entire assembly is then given an impregnation and coating of plastic, resulting in an electrode with superior fatigue-resistance properties. An undesirable feature of the device is that it is constructed from two dissimilar metals. Even though the Elgiloy does not carry any current, both the Elgiloy and the platinum will come into contact with the body fluids because of the porosity of the plastic used as the encapsulant and will therefore be subject to corrosion. The Elgiloy core will be the part that corrodes, thus decreasing the fatigue resistance of the entire lead. Only extended tests will be able to determine if this corrosion is slow enough for the weakening of the lead material to be negligible.

The General Electric Company has also introduced a lead that has a strength-bearing core of one metal and conductors of a different metal; in this case, however, stranded wire is used instead of yarn. This device also trades increased fatigue resistance for increased chance of corrosion.

Two additional weak points in the leads are the places where they are attached to the pacemaker and where they are attached to the heart. Since these points are essentially stationary, they are sites where stresses can build up. Adequate stress relief is of great importance at the pacemaker package, which is both rigid and stationary. One method, used in the Medtronics pacemaker, is to terminate the leads in tapered "bullets," or cones, which are inserted into the plastic and held in place by set screws. These screws are insulated by room-temperature-vulcanizing silicone rubber, which can be applied by the surgeon during the operation. Thus, if the batteries should fail, the pacemaker unit can be changed without replacing the leads. The construction of the lead is such that there is no sudden transition in stiffness. Unfortunately, all pacemakers at the present time must have some provision for replacing the power unit while leaving the leads in place, which considerably complicates the problem of providing adequate stress relief and of obtaining a good seal.

The design of the stress relief at the heart has usually turned out to be somewhat simpler, because no hermetic seal is required here and no rigid connection is needed. The end of the leads are sutured into the heart, and as long as sharp bends and welds are not used there seem to be no particular problems. One difficulty that has arisen has been with the length of electrode penetrating into the heart muscle. The muscle is composed of three layers that move in somewhat different directions. Thus, if the electrode tip is long enough to cross two layers, it will be subjected to large and complex shear and bending forces. This was actually the case with some early electrodes, which frequently broke inside the heart. Limiting the length to about $\frac{1}{4}$ in. seems to have solved this problem.

REFERENCES

[1] Zoll, P. M., "Resuscitation of Heart in Ventricular Standstill by External Electric Stimulation," *New England J. Med.,* 247:768 (1952).

[2] Parsonnet, V., I. R. Zucker, M. Kannerstein, L. Gilbert, and J. Alvares, "The Fate of Permanent Intracardiac Electrodes," *J. Surg. Res.,* 6:285 (1966).

[3] Greatbatch, W., and W. Chardack, "Myocardial and Endocardial Electrodes for Chronic Implantation," *Ann. N. Y. Acad. Sci.,* 148:234 (Art. 1) (1968).

[4] Weinman, J., and H. Mahler, "An Analysis of the Electrical Properties of Metal Electrodes," *Med. Elec. Biol. Eng.,* 2:265 (1964).

[5] Schwan, H. P., "Electrode Polarization Impedance and Measurements in Biological Materials," *Ann. N. Y. Acad. Sci.,* 148:191 (Art. 1) (1968).

[6] Lewin, G., G. H. Myers, V. Parsonnet, and I. R. Zucker, "A Non-Polarizing Electrode for Physiological Stimulation," *Trans. Am. Soc. Artificial Internal Organs,* 13:345 (1967).

CHAPTER SEVEN

Clinical Use of Implanted Pacemakers

At this time the cardiac pacemaker is the best example of a completely implantable active artificial organ. As long ago as 1819 Aldini suggested the use of galvanic current for the treatment of syncope (fainting) [1]. He also described attempts made in the 1770s to try to resuscitate dead people with shocks through the chest—experiments that probably influenced his suggestion. He may very well have concluded that, even though shocks could not revive the dead, they might help those who had fainted. In 1929 Gould [2] reported the first successful restoration of the heartbeat in a patient by electricity; the heart of a baby was stimulated by inserting a needle electrode directly into the myocardium. In 1932 Hyman [3] described a laboratory-built pacemaker intended for clinical application, but there is no record of its clinical use. Probably the first practical application of what we now know as heart pacing was Zoll's method [4] of treating Stokes-Adams attacks in 1954 by electrical stimulation of the heart with electrodes placed on the patient's chest. Implanted pacemakers were introduced in 1958 by Chardack [5] in the United States and Senning [6] in Sweden, independently of each other. Intracardiac (or catheter) electrodes were introduced in 1959 [7, 8]; the triggered, or P wave pacemakers, were first described by Nathan and his co-workers in 1963 [9]. The standby, or demand, pacemakers came into prominence in 1964 [10, 11], although numerous investigators had previously described experimental devices that accomplished the same purpose at an earlier date [12–14]. In the 10 years since pacemakers were first implanted much has been learned about their clinical application, their safety, and the problems involved in their development and testing. This chapter summarizes the more important clinical experience with pacemakers. Additional details may be found in the excellent book by Siddons and Sowton [11].

1. ETIOLOGY OF HEART BLOCK

The primary indication for the use of the cardiac pacemaker is complete heart block. In this situation the normal stimulus for contraction of the ventricles of the heart is interrupted by some process. The ventricles then tend to beat at an independent rate determined by the rhythmicity of certain cells within the muscle of the ventricle. This rate is often too slow to maintain adequate circulation, and the patient therefore often has symptoms of an inadequate cardiac output, such as dizziness, fainting and convulsions (Stokes-Adams syndrome); and impairment of the function of other organs, particularly the brain and kidneys. An artificial pacemaker, then, stimulates the heart to beat at a satisfactory rate, but obviously it does nothing to correct the underlying heart disease.

Heart block is most commonly caused by coronary heart disease,—narrowing and obstruction of the arteries of the heart, and interruption of the normal conduction system. Heart block may follow such conditions as rheumatic fever, diphtheria, a few tropical parasitic diseases, and invasion of the conduction system by tumors. Overdoses of certain drugs, particularly digitalis, and imbalance of the body electrolytes, notably potassium and calcium, may also cause abnormal conduction and heart block. Accidental ligation or destruction of the conduction system may occur during repair of defects between the chambers of the heart. The conduction bundle runs along the edge of many of these defects; and, because it is grossly indistinguishable from normal heart muscle, it may be oversewn during surgical repair of tissue. This accident is now rare. Heart block can also be congenital.

As has been stated, in the adult the etiology of heart block is usually coronary heart disease. There are, however, a number of patients, somewhere between 30 and 40 percent, who exhibit no obvious heart disease at the time of the development of heart block; in fact, many such patients even at autopsy fail to reveal a clear-cut cause for this condition. Careful dissection of the conduction system may reveal fibrous scars interrupting the conduction pathway, but the heart block even in these cases is grossly out of proportion to the magnitude of the changes seen in the heart [15]. It is in such cases that the most dramatic and long-term beneficial results can be obtained by pacing, because the coronary circulation and the muscles of the ventricles are normal.

2.   INDICATIONS FOR PACING

The most important and frequent clinical indication for insertion of the pacemaker is heart block. (Heart block may be complete, in which none of the atrial impulses reach the ventricle; partial or second degree, in which some of the atrial impulses are conducted to the ventricle; or first degree, in which the conduction time from the atrium to the ventricle is merely prolonged.)

Whether or not all patients with complete heart block require a pacemaker remains a medical question, but it is likely that sooner or later all such patients will require a pacemaker. Use of medications alone is usually not sufficient to prevent symptoms, although there are patients who have been treated successfully for many years without pacemakers. More recently, since the safety of implantable pacemakers has been demonstrated, the indications for treatment have been extended to include very slow heart rates. (Sinus bradycardia and various other types of symptomatic bradycardia may occur, as well as intermittent block where sinus rhythms and heart block alternate.) There is a variety of other chaotic arrhythmias that can also be treated with pacemakers, but a discussion of these problems is beyond the scope of this text.

3.   PACING TECHNIQUES

The heart can be stimulated with one or two electrodes in contact with heart-muscle fibers (monopolar and bipolar pacing). For monopolar pacing the stimulating electrode should be the cathode; the anode, or indifferent electrode, is placed in some convenient distant area of the body.

The wires can be brought to the heart in a variety of ways. The first method described was direct insertion of needles through the chest wall into the heart. Electrodes were then threaded through the needle [16]. Subsequently wires were sewn directly into the heart muscle, which had been exposed through a chest incision; and most recently electrodes have been passed through veins and into the chambers of the heart to make contact with the inner surface of the right ventricle [7, 8]. The latter catheter technique is now popular because the operation can be done under local anesthesia with very little risk in critically ill patients.

Pacing of the heart can be *short term* or *long term*. For short-term pacing the pacemaker is used during an acute episode of heart block or during incidental surgery. It is also used as emergency treatment of syncope resulting from complete heart block until the patient is ready for definitive insertion of a permanent pacemaker. Some of these patients may, during the period of temporary pacing, recover from the heart block and never require a permanent unit [17].

Long-term pacing of the heart, although possible with catheters or wires attached to an exterior pacemaker, is usually best performed with an implantable unit.

4. PACEMAKING MODES

The most popular pacemaker to date has been the fixed-rate unit, which produces a stimulus at a predetermined rate irrespective of the behavior of the heart. Since this pacemaker stimulates the heart continually, whether or not the patient's heart returns to regular rhythm, there may be competition between the natural heartbeats and the pacemaker beats. It is possible that such an eventuality can be dangerous, because if the pacemaker impulse reaches the heart during a certain vulnerable period (the apex of the T wave), ventricular fibrillation (a chaotic rhythm of the heart incompatible with life) may occur.

The synchronous pacemaker is in effect an artificial conduction system, because the pacemaker senses the atrial excitation wave that usually continues to occur at a physiologic rate. After a suitable delay, approximately equivalent to a normal PR interval, the pacemaker stimulates the ventricles. In other words, the ventricular contraction is synchronous with the atrial rate. This pacemaker is particularly useful in young patients who require considerable adjustment of the heart rate in response to varying bodily demands. Synchronization of the atrial and ventricular contractions produces the maximum filling of the ventricles and therefore is important in producing optimum cardiac output in patients with borderline ventricular function.* (Ordinarily in patients with fairly strong ventricles the small increment in cardiac output obtained by synchronization is not essential.) Synchronous pacing is also indicated in patients who tend to develop competition, because with synchronization competition is not likely to occur.

The standby (or demand) pacemaker, a more recent development, in effect turns itself off when its use is not required. There are two forms of standby pacemakers available [18]. Both sense the ventricular R wave. In one an R wave that occurs faster than the built-in fixed rate of the pacemaker will block the next electrical stimulus. In the other the R wave signals the pacemaker to fire without delay (a ventricular synchronous pacemaker), so that the electrical stimulus falls in the absolute refractory period of the R wave. The standby pacemaker was designed to solve the problem of competition by

---

*Patients with fixed-rate pacemakers adjust their cardiac output by changing the stroke volume of each heart contraction. When there is a large demand for circulation the stroke volume will increase, and vice versa. Synchronous pacemakers, on the other hand, respond to the increased demand by changing the rate proportional to the physiologic requirements.

turning the pacemaker off whenever an extrasystole or some type of spontaneous rhythm faster than the fixed rate of the pacemaker occurred. There is, as will be shown, rather strong evidence that patients with competition are protected by this mode of pacing.

5. SURGICAL CONSIDERATION FOR PERMANENT IMPLANTS

Originally the most acceptable technique for the insertion of a pacemaker was through an open thoracotomy, in which the chest was entered on the left between the fifth and sixth ribs, the overlying lung was retracted, the pericardium was opened, and wires were inserted directly into the heart muscle. Other methods of approaching the heart have also been described. One of these is to approach the under surface of the heart through an abdominal incision [12]. This method has been used for patients who may not tolerate an opening in the chest. Incisions of many kinds have also been described, including very short ones on the right or left of the sternum, through which wires can be advanced to the heart. Because of the requirements for special skills, these techniques have not become popular.

It is now customary to insert catheter electrodes for permanent pacing [19]. Generally the catheter electrode is inserted through a vein in the neck or beneath the clavicle and positioned in the heart by observing its progress under a fluoroscope. The other end of the lead is attached to the pacemaker, which can be implanted in a convenient position beneath the skin of the chest wall.

No matter what technique is used, the pulse generator (pacemaker) may be placed in almost any accessible position of the body, including the chest within the abdomen, in the armpit, chest wall, abdominal wall, or even in the space behind the abdomen above the kidneys. Experience has shown that the pacemaker is best placed as deeply as possible in the subcutaneous tissues so that there is minimal tendency for the overlying skin to be damaged. The chest is the preferred location because here the wires tend to be splinted by the chest wall, preventing wire fatigue fractures. In our experience there has never been a lead fracture of a helical coil wire in this position except where some type of splicing had been carried out. Pacemakers positioned in the abdomen, on the other hand, have a higher incidence of wire fractures because of the unusual buckling that occurs in sitting, stooping, etc.

6. TYPICAL SURGICAL APPROACH TO INSERTION OF THE PACEMAKER

There are numerous methods of inserting a pacemaker. A typical procedure would be the following: A patient is admitted to the hospital with a slow pulse resulting from complete heart block. He may also have convulsive seizures (Stokes-Adams attacks) because of a reduced cardiac output. As soon as possible after admission the patient is transferred to the catheterization room, where under sterile technique and local anesthesia a temporary bipolar electrode catheter is passed through a vein (usually in the neck) into the right ventricle. The electrodes are connected to an external battery-powered pacemaker, and the heart rate is then immediately controlled. Thereafter, during a period of close observation, a detailed medical evaluation is obtained to ascertain the severity of the patient's disease, the complications that may exist, and to choose the approximate time for permanent implantation of a pacemaker.

When that time has arrived, usually 2 to 7 days later, the patient is taken to the catheterization room, and again under local anesthesia the vein on the opposite side of the chest beneath the clavicle is exposed through a short incision. A unipolar catheter electrode is then advanced (under fluoroscopic control) through the veins and into the apex of the right ventricle, where it is wedged as tightly as possible, but not too forcefully for fear of penetration of the muscle. After satisfactory fluoroscopic positioning has been achieved, the stimulus threshold for the new electrode is tested with a standard laboratory oscilloscope and a battery-powered pacemaker. Usually a stimulus of 0.4 to 0.5 volts and 0.6 to 0.9 ma is adequate for pacing. If the threshold is higher than this, a new position of electrode must be found. Thereafter the pacemaker is attached to the end of the lead, suitable silicone adhesive is placed around the connecting plug, and the pacemaker is placed in a previously prepared deep subcutaneous pocket in the upper chest area. The wound is then closed, and a light dressing is applied.

Patients are usually ambulatory on the following day and are discharged 4 to 7 days later. Immediately after the insertion of the permanent pacemaker the temporary electrode is removed from the vein on the opposite side, and the patient is thereafter no longer encumbered by external devices.

A still popular alternative technique for insertion of the permanent unit is the transthoracic method. Here, after having inserted a temporary electrode as described above, the patient is taken to the operating room where a formal chest operation is performed under general endotracheal anesthesia. The chest is opened between the fifth and sixth ribs, on the left, and the pericardium is opened. Wires are sewn directly into the heart, and the pacemaker is placed usually in the chest wall, but occasionally in the abdominal wall. The wound is closed, and a dry dressing is applied. Usually the chest must be drained for a day or two. Following this type of operation patients are uncomfortable, because chest incisions tend to be painful. However most patients can tolerate this procedure without difficulty.

7. CLINICAL RESULTS

For completeness it would be of some interest to report the results of the authors and their co-workers in the use of permanently implanted pacemakers. There are many pacemaker centers throughout the world with an equivalent experience, and their results are similar. Rather than summarize the information acquired from many other clinics, it seems best to report our own findings of closely observed patients over an 8-year period.

A total of 248 patients have had permanent pacemakers implanted. Of these 162 have been male and 86 have been female, with the mean age for the men of 70 and for the females of 73. These figures are more or less to be expected because they parallel the sex distribution of coronary heart disease. There have been 45 deaths, leaving 203 patients living. The youngest patient in our series was 38 and the oldest 95. There were no children in this group, because of the nature of the hospital in which the work was carried out. Most cases of pediatric and surgical heart block are to be found in centers where pediatric cardiac surgery is performed.

The surgical techniques used by us have been varied. In all but six patients there was preliminary insertion of a temporary bipolar electrode. In these six the clinical situation was so obvious, and the condition of the patient so good, that it was not considered necessary to subject the patient to two procedures. However, this situation is obviously exceptional.

The first 71 patients had standard transthoracic (or the somewhat similar transdiaphragmatic) pacemaker insertion. Since then, with the exception of three cases in which the chest was entered for insertion of synchronous pacemakers, all permanent pacemakers have been inserted by the transvenous tech-

TABLE 1. Mortality Following Pacemaker Implantation

Technique	Complete Operations	Number of Patients	Number of Operative Deaths
Transthoracic (including transdiaphragmatic)	85	74[a]	2(2.5%)
Transvenous	199	174[b]	2(1.0%)
Totals	284	248[c]	4(1.5%)

[a] Including one converted from transvenous and four converted from transthoracic to transdiaphragmatic.
[b] Including 15 converted from transthoracic.
[c] Twenty patients counted twice.

nique. In the former method there were two postoperative deaths in 85 operations (see Table 1).

In the transvenous method, on the other hand, there were two deaths in 199 operations. (Fifteen of the patients with transthoracic pacemakers eventually had replacements with a transvenous pacemaker.) In other words, there was a 1 percent mortality from the transvenous operations as compared with 2.5 percent in the older transthoracic method.

Similarly, operative morbidity has been reduced. Whereas patients with open-chest operations went home in about 14 days following surgery, those with transvenous pacemakers often were ready to go home in 3 or 4 days, but typically were kept in the hospital for 7 days until sutures were removed. There was very little discomfort from the operation with this method, and surgical complications have been mild and easily controlled.

8. MISCELLANEOUS RESULTS

The longest life of a pacemaker was 47 months (an Electrodyne unit). The mean survival time of all pulse generators used, including those that failed in the early series, was 22 months. Most patients needed additional operations between pacemaker changes. On the average patients had 1.4 operations per year. Apart from replacements of decayed pulse generators, other types of operations related to the pacemaker were splicing of broken wires, moving the pacemaker from one site to another because of infection or muscle twitching from proximity of the indifferent electrode to voluntary muscle, and complete replacement of pacemakers because of dislodgement of electrodes from the heart. In addition, patients underwent major operations for other diseases. There were 35 unrelated operations, such as transurethral prostatectomies, bowel resections, gall-bladder operations, and hernia repairs.

Most significantly, patients continued to live despite repeated pacemaker operations, and most patients continued to function well. A detailed survey indicated that most individuals returned to a normal life; many played golf, swam, traveled by air (at least one went around the world), and had sexual intercourse; many returned to their previous occupations.

Despite the apparent severe illness of many individuals before treatment, there was usually dramatic rehabilitation after insertion of the pacemaker. Of the 10 patients operated on in the first year (1961), seven are still alive. All seven have had repeated operations during the ensuing seven years, but all continue to function happily. Of the remaining group there was approximately 10 percent decay per year in the patient population. This parallels closely the expected mortality of patients without heart block in this age group.

TABLE 2. Incidence of Sudden Deaths in Pacemaker Implants

	Fixed Rate		Standby	
	Patients	Deaths	Patients	Deaths
Competition	24	9	65[a]	1
No competition	62	1	21	0
Total	86	10	86	1

[a] Including three Atricor (synchronous pacemakers).

The patients that died usually did so from other causes. Of the 45 deaths, 34 resulted from miscellaneous diseases such as stroke, gastrointestinal hemorrhage, cancer, and congestive heart failure. There were 11 sudden deaths, most of which could not be explained satisfactorily (see Table 2).

It has been maintained by some that there is no danger to the patient when competition between idiocardiac contractions and a fixed-rate pacemaker occur. In fact, in laboratory studies we have been unable to demonstrate significant arrhythmias from competitive pacing unless the heart is altered in some way by various drugs and anoxia [20]. Although at most times the paced human heart may be relatively insensitive to competition, the fibrillation threshold may be lowered by anoxia, digitalis toxicity, electrolyte imbalance, and other factors. In these situations competition can become dangerous. In fact, repetitive rhythms [21] and ventricular fibrillation [22] have been documented in humans following stimulation of the heart in its vulnerable period by a standard pacemaker stimulus.

Almost every report of studies throughout the world of large groups of patients with pacemakers has mentioned a few unaccountable sudden deaths. Similarly 11 sudden deaths have occurred in our patients, most of them having fixed-rate pacemaker and competition. Such striking differences in mortality between patients with fixed-rate and standby pacing have convinced the authors that, in general, fixed-rate pacemakers should not be used except as a replacement in cases that have shown no evidence of competition for several years.

REFERENCES

[1] Albert, H. M., B. A. Glass, J. A. Andonie, and K. C. Cranor, "Pacemaker Failure in Complete Heart Block," *Circ. Res.*, 10:295 (1962).
[2] Gould, Medical Congress, Sidney, Australia; cited by Hyman, A. S., "Resuscitation of the Stopped Heart by Intracardial Therapy," *Arch. Intern. Med.*, 50:283 (1932).
[3] Hyman, A. S., "Resuscitation of the Stopped Heart by Intracardial Therapy," *Arch. Intern. Med.*, 50:283 (1932).

[4] Zoll, P. M., "Resuscitation of the Heart in Ventricular Standstill by External Electric Stimulation," *New England J. Med.,* 247:768 (1952).

[5] Greatbatch, W., and W. M. Chardack, "A Transistorized Implantable Pacemaker for the Long-Term Correction of Complete Atrioventricular Block," *Med. Electron. NEREM,* 8 (1959).

[6] Senning, A., in discussion, *J. Thorac. Cardiovasc. Surg.,* 38:639 (1959).

[7] Furman, S., and G. Robinson, "The Use of an Intracardiac Pacemaker in the Correction of Total Heart Block," *Surg. Forum,* 9:245 (1958).

[8] Parsonnet, V., I. R. Zucker, L. Gilbert, and M. Asa, "An Intracardiac Bipolar Electrode for Interim Treatment of Complete Heart Block," *Amer. J. Cardiol.,* 10:261 (1962).

[9] Nathan, D. A., S. Center, C-Y Wu, W. Keller, "An Implantable Synchronous Pacemaker for the Long-Term Correction of Complete Heart Block," *Amer. J. Cardiol.,* 11:362 (1963).

[10] Parsonnet, V., I. R. Zucker, G. H. Myers, J. W. Keller, Jr., and L. Gilbert, "An Implantable Permanent Transvenous Standby Pacemaker" (abstract), *Clinical Research,* 13:527 (1965).

[11] Siddons, H., and E. Sowton, *Cardiac Pacemakers,* Thomas, Springfield, Ill., (1962).

[12] Nicks, R., G. F. H. Stening, and E. C. Hulme, "Some Observations on the Surgical Treatment of Heart Block in Degenerative Heart Disease," *Med. J. Aust.,* 49(2):857 (1962).

[13] Effert, S., H. J. Sykosch, and K. G. Pulver, "Langfristige Therapie mit implantierbaren elektrischen Schrittmachern," *Deutsch. Med. Wschr.,* 89:654 (1964).

[14] Lemberg, L., A. Castellanos, and B. V. Berkovits, "Pacemaking on Demand in A.V. Block," *JAMA,* 191:12 (1965).

[15] Parsonnet, V., L. Gilbert, I. R. Zucker, and I. Assefi, "Subcostal Transdiaphragmatic Insertion of a Cardiac Pacemaker," *J. Thorac. Cardiovasc. Surg.,* 49:739 (1965).

[16] Weirich, W. L., V. L. Gott, and C. W. Lillehei, "The Treatment of Complete Heart Block by the Combined Use of a Myocardial Electrode and an Artificial Pacemaker," *Surg. Forum,* 8:360 (1957).

[17] Parsonnet, V., I. R. Zucker, L. Gilbert, E. L. Rothfeld, D. K. Brief, and J. Alpert, "An Evaluation of Transvenous Pacing of the Heart in Complete Heart Block Following Acute Myocardial Infarction," *Israel J. Med. Sciences,* Vol. 3, 2:306 (1967).

[18] Parsonnet, V., I. R. Zucker, L. Gilbert, E. L. Rothfeld, J. Alpert, and D. K. Brief, "Clinical Experience with Implanted Standby Pacemakers," *Surgery,* 63:188 (1968).

[19] Parsonnet, V., I. R. Zucker, L. Gilbert, D. K. Brief, and J. Alpert, "Permanent Transvenous Pacing of the Heart," *Israel J. Med. Sciences,* Vol. 3, 5:210 (1967).

[20] Zucker, I. R., E. L. Rothfeld, V. Parsonnet, L. Gilbert, and A. Bernstein, "Competitive Idiocardiac and Extrinsic Pacemaker Stimuli in Heart Block," *Am. Heart J.,* 69:62 (1965).

[21] Chardack, W. M., "A Myocardial Electrode for Long-Term Pacemaking," *Ann. N. Y. Acad. Sci.,* 111:893 (1964).

[22] Bilitch, M., R. S. Cosby, and E. A. Cafferky, "Competition as Mortality Factor in Asynchronous Cardiac Pacing," *Am. J. Cardiol.,* 19:120 (1967).

CHAPTER EIGHT

Materials in the Body

1. PLASTIC MATERIALS IN THE BODY

Some of the problems that arose in the early development and application of the pacemaker are typical of those that have arisen with numerous other artificial internal organs. The basic concept of the device was clear, and it could be proved to work in short-term experiments. After long-term implantation, however, problems with the materials used began to arise. This pattern has repeated itself with so many devices, including artificial hearts, artificial heart valves, and artificial kidneys, in addition to the pacemaker, that it seems fair to say that a major problem that will be encountered in the development of implanted devices is the discovery and application of suitable materials both for construction and for implantation. Unfortunately, this is a problem that is difficult to analyze and solve, because many of the faults do not appear until after a considerable period of time and, by definition, only after implantation in living tissues. The difficulty is compounded by the problem of obtaining statistically significant data in the face of all of the variables that may appear in living creatures. This section and the following attempt to summarize some of the published knowledge on materials in the body, primarily as they relate to implanted organs of the type represented by pacemakers (or other implanted electronic devices) or artificial hearts and other mechanical devices. Load-bearing problems, such as are encountered with all types of artificial bones, will not be considered as a separate topic.

There are six basic problems that must be solved in selecting an implanted material:

1. The material must have sufficient strength.
2. It must have a long life without appreciable degradation of its properties.
3. It must be compatible with the body tissues.
4. It must not be carcinogenic.
5. It must not damage blood, which could occur if the blood cells were destroyed (hemolysis), if the proteins became denatured, or if clots were formed.

6. In the case of encapsulated devices it must be waterproof.

Needless to say, there is no single material that meets all of these requirements, and so compromises are always necessary. Platinum has been widely used, and it comes close to meeting many of these needs; however, platinum, besides being extremely expensive, is difficult to fabricate for many of the applications in which it might be used.

Medical Silicones

Medical-grade silicone rubber [1, 2] has undoubtedly been one of the most successful plastics used inside the human body, because it is inert and causes almost no tissue reaction. It is also flexible and easily fabricated. However, it is not as strong as some other materials and in comparison with many other plastics it is permeable to water vapor.

All silicones are polymers, long chains composed of many repetitions of a basic building block. However, unlike organic polymers where the links are carbon atoms, the silicones are made of chains of alternating silicon and oxygen atoms, as illustrated in Figure 8.1. Two organic groups are usually attached to each silicone atom, the most common being methyl, CH_3, as is shown in the figure. Also used are phenyl groups, C_6H_5, and vinyl groups, C_2H_3, as well as fluorinated aliphatic groups in some special cases. Because the majority of the silicones have mainly methyl groups, they are sometimes generically (and somewhat erroneously) referred to as the polydimethylsiloxanes.

A *siliconized* surface is one that has been treated with a silicone, much as a board is painted or any other surface is treated. Siliconizing does not change the substrate, so a piece of siliconized rubber or plastic is not necessarily suitable for implanting just because it has received this treatment; silicone rubber and siliconized rubber are completely different materials. Note that silicone rubber contains no natural rubber—a better name would be silicone elastomer. Most medical experience has been with silicone rubber, although other forms have been used in various applications.

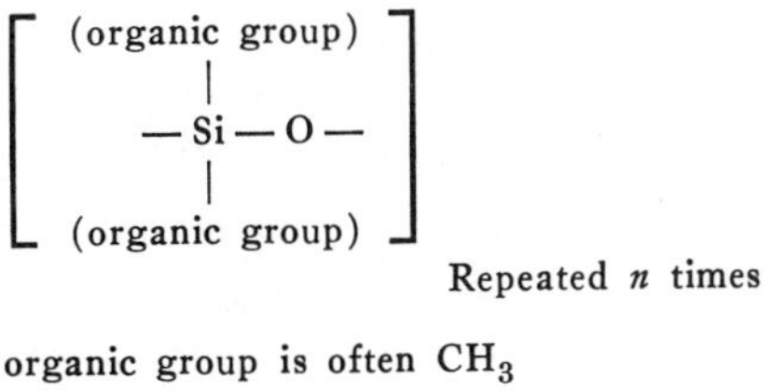

$$\left[\begin{array}{c} \text{(organic group)} \\ | \\ -\,Si\,-\,O\,- \\ | \\ \text{(organic group)} \end{array} \right]$$

Repeated n times

The organic group is often CH_3

Figure 8.1 Diagram showing composition of silicones.

Property	Value
Dielectric strength	450-600 V/mil
Dielectric constant	2.9 to 3.6
Dissipation factor	5×10^{-4} to 2×10^{-2}
Volume resistivity	10^{13} to 10^{15} ohm cm

Dielectric strength measured with 1/4-in. electrodes on specimen 1/16-in. thick. (After Braley.)

Figure 8.2 Typical electrical properties of silicone rubber.

Silicone fluids are the simplest types of silicones. They can have viscosities as low as that of ether or so high that they are solid. Their chemical nature can be changed by substituting other organic radicals for some of the methyl groups. Silicone rubber is made from the high-viscosity fluids. There are two major types: heat-vulcanizing forms and room-temperature-vulcanizing forms. The heat-vulcanizing type is like modeling clay in its raw state, but the vulcanized final product is tough and strong. The room-temperature-vulcanizing (RTV) silicone rubbers are liquid in the raw state. All of the medical grades are vulcanized by stannous octoate, which is stirred in by the user. Vulcanization takes place within a few minutes. Typical physical and electrical properties of the two types of rubber are shown in Figures 8.2 and 8.3.

A special room-temperature-vulcanizing silicone rubber is used medically as an adhesive. It has the consistency of Vaseline in its raw state and sets up by reaction with water vapor in the environment. It is used as a glue or sealant would be used. It adheres to many other materials besides silicone rubber, but it does not adhere well to tissue, certain plastics, or unetched Teflon.

The principal advantages of the medical-grade silicone rubbers in the body are the following:

1. Heat Stability. The silicones can be sterilized repeatedly by autoclaving or by dry heat without damage.

2. No Adherence. Nothing will adhere to a silicone except another sili-

Property	Heat-Vulcanizing Type	Room-Temperature (RTV) Type Vulcanizing
Durometer	30-80	50-60
Tensile strength	1000 psi	500 psi
Elongation	300%	150%

(After Braley.)

Figure 8.3 Typical physical properties of silicone rubber.

cone, and the body will not grow onto it; clots, urinary stones, drainage fluid, and other internal substances will not adhere. Because of the dielectric properties of the elastomer, however, it may develop a surface charge and hold dust and lint. If adhesion to tissue is desired, it can be accomplished by attaching the silicone to an artificial foundation of Dacron or Teflon cloth. Tissue growing into this will anchor the silicone part in place.

3. No Change with Time. In general properly cured silicone rubbers do not show any effects of degradation with time when implanted in the body. Recently, changes have been noted in some artificial valves after considerable periods of time, but it is not known whether this was caused by improper preparation or is related to the basic properties of the silicone rubber.

4. Lack of Foreign Body Reaction. A properly prepared medical-grade silicone rubber causes the formation of a thin, delicate fibrous-tissue (scar tissue) membrane around it but no inflammation reaction. However, when tissue is stretched over a sharp or rough implant, inflammation can occur, so surface preparation is extremely important.

Perhaps the outstanding disadvantage of the silicone rubber is its permeability and porosity. In fact, this property has been exploited in an experimental chemical pacemaker, in which a cardiac stimulant was placed in a silicone-rubber capsule and implanted in the heart [3]. The material gradually leached out, and stimulated the heart. A device encapsulated in silicone rubber will eventually have moisture on its inside. Moreover, this is true of all plastics—including the epoxy resins, which are used to encapsulate many current pacemakers and which are commonly considered impervious. Because moisture passes through the encapsulating material it has been necessary to ensure that all metals inside the pacemaker are electrolytically compatible (including all of the leads). Otherwise electrolytic corrosion occurs inside the case, leading to lead breakage and component failure.* Great care must also be taken in the encapsulation process to ensure that no air bubbles are present in the plastics. This can be done by placing the molds under a vacuum before the plastics have cured. A common procedure for using plastics to encapsulate implanted electronics is to first encase the device in a material with mechanical properties that are superior to those of the silicones, such as epoxy resins or Teflon, and then to encase the entire device in silicone rubber. Teflon, unfortunately, has a high curing temperature (700°F), which precludes its use in many applications.

Surface characteristics are of great importance when the possibility of clot formation exists, such as in artificial blood vessels or in the artificial heart. In the past it was always assumed that any object placed in the blood stream

* E. Bakken, personal communication.

should have a highly polished surface, so that blood elements would not adhere to it and form clots [4]. However, when a polished surface is next to tissue, the tissue at the interface provides an anchor for streamers of clot that temporarily adhere to the adjacent smooth surface, proliferate, and then separate from the smooth surface. More clot then forms in the gap between the flap of clot anchored to the tissue and the underlying smooth material. This process continues until portions of the clot are too large to be supported by the delicate tissue anchor. As a result, they break off and block the blood vessel (form an embolus). If the tissue holds, the clot may spread and still block the blood vessel (or, in the case of the heart, interfere with the operation of a valve). The silicone rubber ball of the ball-in-cage type of heart valve has no interface and rotates in its cage. These factors combine to inhibit clots. It is only in this application that extreme smoothness and inertness are important.

Paradoxically, a rough surface produces a layer of fibrous tissue that does not break off because it becomes entrapped in the interstices of the surface. This natural body tissue forms a new lining that does not promote clot formation when used, for example, as an artificial blood vessel. In very narrow vessels, however, even this layer is a problem because the diameter of the vessel decreases somewhat and, if it is small enough to begin with, complete occlusion of the lumen will occur. The large blood vessels turn out to be the most crucial ones in clinical practice, and in these rough surfaces effectively solve the clotting problems.

Other Plastics and Tissue Compatibility

Although silicone rubber is probably the most widely used plastic in the human body, others have found application, such as Teflon, epoxy resins, nylon, Dacron, polyvinyls, polyurethanes, and polyethylenes. [2] These all have advantages in certain applications as far as their chemical, physical, and mechanical properties are concerned; for example, polymethylmethacrylate turns out to be well suited for the artificial cornea, and Dacron has been the most widely used plastic for artificial blood vessels. The question of whether a material's properties are suitable for one application or another will not be discussed here.

In discussing compatibility we must consider resistance to degradation, changes in properties during implantation, foreign-body reactions, and destruction of red blood cells (hemolysis).

Degradation. There are three principal factors that contribute to the degradation of organic polymers under the influence of the numerous chemical reagents present in the body:

1. Chemical bonds that may react with the body constituents and eventually be severed by this action.

2. Atoms or groups near these bonds that either activate or protect them.

3. The supermolecular character of the polymer (oriented, amorphous, crystalline, folded, cross-linked, etc.), which does not affect the intrinsic chemical reactivity of the sensitive bonds but affects their accessibility to outside influences and therefore their susceptibility to degradation.

The chemical reagents that may cause degradation include acids, bases, oxygen (or ozone), and microorganisms or enzymes, all of which may be found in the body. The types of chemical bond that react with these ingredients and may be found in the polymers likely to be used are C—O, C—S, C—N, C=N, C=C, and Si—O. By contrast, C—C is much more difficult to attack. The types of atom or groups that may be in proximity to them and may affect the properties of the materials are principally F, Cl, OH, NH_2, COOH, CH_3, and CF_3. There are undoubtedly others that also have an effect.

The effects just described, which belong under the first two categories, are mainly chemical. There are still the physical effects, which belong under the third category. These are basically related to the crystallinity of the substance. Crystallization is a physical effect that is strongly influenced by physical processes such as orientation, seeding, and swelling. The degree of crystallinity affects swelling characteristics, rate of take up of swelling agents, and ultimate amount of material. Highly crystalline material does not degrade; only the amorphous portion degrades, leaving the crystalline part.

Cross-linking must also be considered. It has long been known that favorable properties can be obtained by the chemical cross-linking of long flexible-chain molecules. A good example is rubber. As more and more cross-links are introduced, their average distance along the flexible chains decreases, and the system is progressively stiffened until we finally have hard rubber, or Ebonite —a material that is rigid, has a high softening range, and is completely insoluble and stable. By suitable manipulation of cross-linking and crystallinity it is possible also to control degradation.

Changes During Implantation. In spite of the fact that plastics have been used in humans for a number of years, there is surprisingly little information in the literature on the effect of the body on the plastics. The determination of the changes in properties of a plastic as an implant is simple in theory, but in practice there are many difficulties, which may account for much of the scarcity of data. Because most research must be done in animals, there is the possibility that different species will produce different effects. The location is

Material	Days Implanted	Percent Loss of Tensile Strength
Nylon	1073	80.7
Dacron	780	11.4
Orlon	735	23.8
	670	1.0
Teflon	677	5.3
	675	7.0

Figure 8.4   Changes in tensile strength of plastic after implantation. (After Leininger.)

also important, because, for example, a muscle implant has different environmental characteristics than a blood vessel. Also, the statistical aspects of the program are difficult especially in obtaining a significant sample for each property to be measured. The American Society for Testing Materials is considering this problem, but at the moment the situation is up to each individual investigator. The data presented here were collected by Leininger [5]; a new journal, *Journal of Biomedical Materials,** many add much useful information for the future.

In one of the earliest studies [5] fabric grafts of nylon, Dacron, Orlon, Teflon, Vinyon, and polyethylene were implanted in dogs to replace portions of the descending thoracic aorta. Figure 8.4 shows the changes measured after implantation, and it can be seen that nylon lost most of its strength in 3 years; whereas the others lost measurable, but not large amounts, in 2 years.

In tests by another investigator [6] a thermoplastic polyurethane was implanted intramuscularly in dogs. The specimens were in the form of strips 9 cm long by 0.2 mm thick. Figure 8.5 shows the extreme loss in tensile strength of this material in the first 8 months. Within 16 months the samples had disintegrated so much that tensile strengths could not be measured. The results indicated that the breaking of the polymer chains had taken place through hydrolysis.

In Leininger's laboratory films of five plastics [5] were implanted intra-

Time in Months	Tensile Strength (psi)
0	8150
8	1846
16	Disintegrated

Figure 8.5   Changes in properties of polyurethane. (After Harrison.)

* Interscience Publishers.

Material	Tensile Strength (psi)		Elongation (%)	
	Control	17 Months	Control	17 Months
Polyethylene	2,700	1,930	780	420
Teflon	2,950	3,720	320	250
Mylar	18,300	18,440	100	100
Nylon	9,300	5,200	550	140
Silastic	950	930	800	890

Figure 8.6   Changes in properties of some plastic cylinders after implantation. (After Leininger.)

muscularly in the flank of dogs. The materials were 4-mil polyethylene, 5-mil Teflon, 5-mil Mylar type A, 10-mil nylon, and 5-mil Silastic (trade name for silicone rubber) X30146. In each case five samples of the film were removed after 6, 11, and 17 months of implantation, and the changes in tensile strength and elongation to break were measured. The results are shown in Figure 8.6. The changes in Silastic and Mylar are not significant, but the increase in tensile strength for Teflon may be significant. The fact that the elongation also decreased may indicate an increase in brittleness. Polyethylene has probably had its chains split, ending up with a lower molecular weight, and nylon has degraded even further.

The small amount of available information on the fate of plastics used as implants makes it clear that much more work must be done in this area if plastics resistant to the body environment are to be developed.

Compatibility. The subject of "compatibility" includes local tissue responses caused by implanted material, toxic effect, production of antibodies, and carcinogenesis. A review of some of the experiments that have been performed is given, but it should be noted that there have been few studies in which highly reactive materials can be compared quantitatively. The following basic principles are noteworthy:

1. Compatibility tests should mimic as closely as possible the actual application in relation to physical form, test subject, and site of implantation; for example, injection under the skin of animals of polyvinyl alcohol, a high-molecular-weight polymer, may produce high blood pressure; on the other hand, the same material fabricated into a sponge can be used successfully as an implant in man.

2. The complex nature of the responses indicates that animal testing must be followed by human testing. Most internal devices currently in use have been developed this way. Man and test animals may differ significantly in their responses to implanted materials.

3. The results of tissue damage from the implant are not the same at all sites; for example, destruction of nerve cells of the nervous system is permanent, whereas the surface layer of cells of the skin or the gastrointestinal tract has a high rate of regeneration.

4. Polymeric materials that are stable in their usual environment may be chemically altered after implantation, as discussed in the section on degradability. Such changes, which may take a long time to occur, may be the most significant causes of reactions.

5. A nonabsorbed plastic implant may in many circumstances take on some of the aspects of a foreign body with time, and ultimately its original function may disappear; for example, an abdominal wall suture, long after its function as a tissue splint has been fulfilled, may be associated with the development of a foreign-body reaction and may produce sinus tracts to the skin.

A topic of considerable importance is tumor induction (carcinogenesis). The first report of tumors at the sites of polymer implants was by Turner [7], who observed in 1941 that Bakelite films coated with carcinogenic substances caused tumors in rats. Later Oppenheimer [8] observed the development of cancers about cellophane films that had been wrapped around the kidneys of rats to produce artificial hypertension. He also showed that malignant tumors could be produced by subcutaneous implantation of cellophane films in rats. To date tumor induction by this method has been limited to rats, mice, and hamsters and has not been reported for primates or dogs. A lower rate of tumor formation was seen in hamsters, and mice than in rats, in which yields of up to 75 percent have been produced in certain circumstances. At first it was thought that impurities in the materials were responsible for the tumors, but later it was shown that pure cellophane and polyethylene had the same properties. Free-radical initiators were eliminated from consideration as possible causes when they were proved to be noncarcinogenic by themselves, but free-radical breakdown products of the polymer were thought to have possible significance. Materials that have been used to induce subcutaneous tumors in rodents include plastics (usually films) consisting of polyethylene, nylon, Dacron, Teflon, polystyrene, and cellulose hydrate; metals including silver, steel, gold, and liquid mercury; and glass cover slips. Any common chemical mechanism for tumor induction by this variety of substances is certainly obscure.

The incidence of these tumors is related to the size and shape of the implant. Alexander and Horning [9] used squares of Visking sausage casing in rats to show that larger films resulted in a more rapid development and a higher frequency of tumors than did smaller films. With 2 cm squares, over half of the test animals developed tumors in an average of 78 weeks. With a 0.5 cm square, 106 weeks were required for one animal to develop a tumor.

Nonporous films have been shown to be more potent tumor inducers than porous ones. If the test material is implanted as a textile or powder it seems to be less carcinogenic. When the materials are made into Millipore filters, reduction of pore size from 450 to 50 millimicrons (or increase in surface area) was associated with an increased incidence of tumors.

The tissue response at the implant site has received much study. No tumor develops if the film is removed before 6 months, but tumor formation is independent of the film's presence after 6 months. A foreign-body reaction in which cells align themselves parallel to the film appears during the early months. Afterwards such activity appears to decrease, but not to disappear entirely.

At present the consequences of these experiments for man is not clear. Some of the questions that must be answered are the following:

1. Should prostheses be open networks?

2. How are latent periods for man and rodents compared? The 6-month period in the rat is about one-sixth of his total life. Should this be compared to 10 or 15 years in man? Or, since the time required for wound healing and collagen (scar tissue) formation in man and rat are similar, can any prosthesis be considered safe (noncarcinogenic) in man after 6 months?

3. What circumstances account for tumor induction in the rat, mouse, and hamster that are not present in the guinea pig and, apparently, in man?

4. Should testing of potentially carcinogenic substances rely so heavily on rodents, in view of the obvious differences that have just been discussed?

The polymers just discussed produced tumors after a fairly substantial period of time, but they produced no actual tissue damage at the implanted site. Other polymers, unlike these, are irritating at their implantation sites and can cause considerable local tissue damage that interferes with healing. Techniques to evaluate such damage were described in the study of cyanoacrylate tissue adhesives by Woodward and his associates [10].

Cyanoacrylate tissue adhesives are possible substitutes for existing wound-closure methods. The methods used in comparing the effects of methyl, hexyl, and decyl 2-cyanoacrylate on collagen formation were the following: Under ether anesthesia four sponges were aseptically implanted into pockets created in the four quarters of the abdominal wall. The material used was Eastman 910 (E–910). Before implantation the left-side sponges, which were the controls, were moistened with 0.9 percent saline. The right-side sponges were weighed under sterile conditions before and after impregnation with 5 drops of cyanoacrylate monomer, which diffused evenly throughout the sponge and remained liquid until after implantation. At sacrifice 7 to 28 days later the upper sponge pair was used as controls with respect to weight and hydroxy-

Measurement (Unless noted, units are mg/100 mg dry implanted sponge)	7 Days		14 Days		28 Days	
	E-910	Control	E-910	Control	E-910	Control
Initial sponge wt, mg	30.2	30.5	30.2	30.4	30.2	30.6
E-910 added	540	0	515	0	518	0
Final wet sponge weight	1616	1021	1503	886	1527	860
Final dry sponge weight	657	162	624	186	594	197
Water content	957	859	888	699	934	663
Hydroxyproline content (mg/100 mg dry implanted sponge)	16.9	115	945	1862	1294	2201
Wet tissue weight	947	916	885	785	906	760
Dry tissue weight	9.9	62	8.6	86	—17.5	97
Hydroxyproline concentration (mcg/100 mg dry tissue)	—	2.7	—	2.5	—	21.6
Weight of cyanoacrylate lost	316	0	27.8	0	87	0

Figure 8.7 Changes in impregnated Ivalon sponge implant in the rat (all the values expressed as mean). (After Woodward.)

proline content (which is found to be related to collagen content). The lower sponges were examined by microscope. Sponges were weighed immediately after removal (wet weight), and after drying in a vacuum (dry weight) [10].

Figure 8.7 shows the results of such a study [10]. The collagen, which was estimated from the hydroxyproline, provides most of the tensile strength of a healing wound, so suppression of its growth by a wound-closure adhesive is considered undesirable. The greater water content of the experimental sponges over the control sponges shows that the experimental sponges were not made impermeable by the plastic. An interesting fact is that cyanoacrylate was lost from the implant.

The marked suppression of collagen in the polyvinyl sponge was substantiated by microscopic examination. Figure 8.7 shows that E–910 inhibited collagen [10] growth more in the early period than in the later one. This suggests that either a toxic fraction or product of the polymer was present at first in the implant site, or that young granulation tissue is more sensitive to E–910 than older granulation tissue.

Granulation tissue is new tissue growth, such as might be seen in the small fleshy projections formed on the surface of a gaping wound. Each granula-

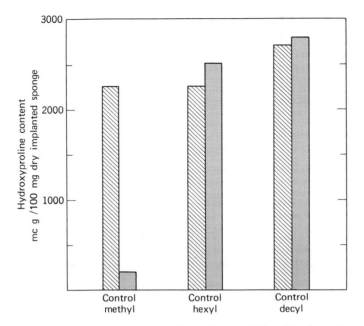

Figure 8.8   Changes in Ivalon sponge implants in rats. (After Woodward.)

tion represents in part the outgrowth of new capillaries by budding from the existing capillaries, interconnection of capillary loops, and proliferation of new connective tissue, all of which will later become fibrous scar tissue. The granulations bring a rich blood supply to the healing surface.

The experimental model just described was used to compare the toxicity of the three types of cyanoacrylates (methyl, hexyl, and decyl), and the results are summarized in Figure 8.8. It is apparent that hexyl and decyl compounds did not suppress growth of collagen in sponges. Unlike methyl sponges, which were almost devoid of granulation tissue and intensely inflamed, hexyl and decyl sponges were infiltrated with granulation tissue and closely resembled their controls.

This study of Woodward points out some of the complexities of the biological evaluations of polymer implants. Methyl 2-cyanoacrylate is soluble only in a very limited number of organic solvents, but it appears to be highly reactive in the body. It is not known whether it is chemically degraded or only physically dispersed from its implant site. The mild inflammatory responses to the other forms suggests that structure-activity relationships that are similar to those developed for some drugs also apply to polymer implants.

A problem of equal importance is the effects of implanted devices on the blood, especially red cell damage, or hemolysis. In particular, mechanical devices such as artificial heart valves and an artificial heart cause hemolysis by mechanical damage to the cell from abnormal velocity, turbulence, and actual crushing of cells in the pump. Although the mechanism of mechanical damage to the red cells is partly understood, many questions are still unanswered. No clinical problems have arisen that suggest any direct effect of implants on white cells. Platelet destruction has been observed in extracorporeal circulation, but no direct chemical effects of implanted materials on the red cells have been identified, unlike the situation with the surrounding tissues.

In addition to red cell destruction, clot (thrombus) formation is a problem with all devices that are in blood vessels. This, of course, includes the artificial heart and artificial valves. Here, too, mechanical problems of flow seem to be significant. Areas of low pressure and stagnation of flow lead to thrombosis. It would seem that the surface properties are important, as already described under the discussion of surface roughness, but a problem here is that *in vitro* tests correlate poorly with those made *in vivo*.

A number of cases of hemolysis have been reported with implanted valves [11–13] and also some in the limited attempts to use heart pumps for prolonged periods of time. Attempts to relate the hemolysis directly to the prosthetic materials used in vitro have so far been unsuccessful, but the number of studies has been limited. Also, in at least two cases where hemolysis developed the implanted device was covered with a layer of tissue, so that the synthetic was not in contact with the blood. Since a variety of materials have been involved in the actual human implants, including Stellite, Lucite, Teflon, Dacron, and silicone rubber, it seems likely that the material itself has very little effect. Only the aortic valve, among valve prostheses, has been incriminated so far in hemolysis. Whereas this may not only be because of the limited number of cases, it is a fact that the blood passing the aortic valve is subjected to a higher pressure gradient and velocity than at the mitral valve, and therefore the possibility of abnormal turbulence is greater. Velocity of flow may also be important. In all of the cases in which significant hemolysis was reported blood was presumably forced at high pressure by the left ventricle through a restricted valve orifice, which would produce great velocity and turbulence. It is not clear whether a rigid inelastic surface is also necessary for red cell destruction. The lack of apparent hemolysis in many patients with artificial devices suggests that the elasticity of the surface itself is not a sufficient explanation.

Destruction of red blood cells has been a significant problem to those designing and using artificial heart-lung machines, and the results of their studies may also be applicable to patients with other types of cardiac prostheses.

A number of types of pumps have been tested for their damaging effects on red cells, but the factors that have led to broad differences between them are not clear. Cahill and Kolff (quoted in Reference 11) suggested that finger-type peristaltic pumps and roller pumps cause injury by crushing red blood cells, causing eddies in the blood and producing local suction. Mc-Caughan (quoted in Reference 11) compared occlusive pumps (which completely block flow during part of the pumping cycle) with nonocclusive pumps and found that hemolysis was less at a given rate of flow when the pump was nonocclusive. Hodges concluded that the stroke volume of a pump is the most significant factor and should be maximized in order to reduce hemolysis. Of course, this may just be because a pump with a large stroke volume has less fluid in contact with its surfaces.

Most investigators agree that red cell destruction is minimized when connections in the device external to the body are smooth and changes in diameters of conduits are achieved by gradual tapering. Stewart and Sturbridge studied the destructive action of tubing on red cells flowing through it. They found that increasing the number of connections increased hemolysis, as did increasing the velocity of the flow. When the tube diameter was doubled flow velocity could be doubled, and rate of flow increased eight times without increasing red cell destruction. Hemolysis was decreased by increasing concentrations of heparin in the blood and also by using tubes with smooth surfaces. Hirose described differences in the amount of hemolysis produced in tubing made from different plastics and noted increased hemolysis after ethylene oxide sterilization, often used for devices containing electronics because it does not require high temperatures (cold sterilization). Bubble oxygenators have caused significant hemolysis, lending more support to the idea of strictly mechanical causes because of the large amount of turbulence and foaming with these devices.

Heart-lung machines also have an intracardiac suction apparatus to remove the blood returned from the coronary and bronchial circulations, and these suction systems have been incriminated as a major source of hemolysis in several studies. It has been reported that when suction pressures were controlled so as to avoid the high pressures that can occur with partial occlusion of the suction line (the occlusion caused by, for example, a suction tip sticking to a surface), hemolysis was markedly diminished. It has also been shown that hemolysis was accentuated when blood and air were drawn through the suction system together.

Thrombosis has presented many problems to those using implantable plastics. This is particularly severe with valves and pumps, where surfaces or moving parts are in the direct path of blood flow. On the other hand, synthetic materials have been used to patch atrial or ventricular defects and as tubes in arterial grafts. Observations in experimental animals have shown that a Teflon patch, or graft, becomes covered by a thin layer of new tissue. The deposit of a thin layer of fibrin (clot material) over the implanted material is a preliminary to the growth of a new membrane over it; ordinarily this fibrin layer will not build up to the point where any damage is done. This modified form of clotting is a desirable stage in the incorporation of the implanted material into normally functioning tissue.

In artificial cardiac valves the problem is to prevent the clot formation that usually begins at the line of attachment of the valve to the heart. The clot may then spread out into the valve, where it can either block the blood flow or break off and form an embolus, which can then travel through the bloodstream and eventually cause blockage of an artery. Thrombosis tends to occur in low pressure areas or where there is stagnation of flow; areas of turbulence, such as at a valve rim or the interior of an aneurysm, also cause clotting. It is strange that none of the patients with hemolysis due to the turbulence of intracardiac prosthetics had any significant clotting about the devices, but this was probably a function of time. Hemolysis is a relatively fast process when compared to intravascular clotting. Thrombosis is more common in mitral than in aortic valve replacements, probably because of the lower pressures and greater opportunity for stagnation about the mitral valve.

Platelets are round or oval disks, formed elements of the blood, that are about 2 to 4 μ in diameter (about one-half the size of a red blood cell); they perform perhaps the most important role in clotting by participating in the mesh of fibrin and red cells, and releasing thromboplastin, which initiates blood clotting. There is evidence to indicate that intracardiac devices do cause platelet destruction, but if so the rate of destruction does not exceed the body's ability to replace them.

Clotting Mechanisms

As a result of applications of new theories of clot prevention, advances in the applications of materials in internal organs may be expected. Some of these theories are discussed here.

All presently known polymers tend to cause blood clotting. However, it is possible to use certain types of surface treatments that will considerably reduce the rate of clot formation, aside from considerations such as the roughness of the surface that have been already mentioned. There is considerable variation in the rate of clot formation depending on the nature of the polymer. The factors that influence this rate are of considerable interest [14].

Lampert in 1930 suggested that the clotting activity of a surface was directly related to its wettability (Lampert's rule); for example, glass is highly wettable and induces clotting much more readily than does paraffin. Although this rule is generally true, there are many exceptions; it gradually became apparent that the relationship was quite complex [14].

A more quantitative approach to the relationship between wettability and clot formation was developed by Lyman [16], who showed that a rough correlation existed between the log of the surface free energy and the clotting time. Silicone rubber, however, has a very low surface free energy and still causes clotting. It has been shown that most foreign surfaces adsorb proteins from the blood, so the surface presented to the blood is actually not the plastic at all.

The electrical charge of a surface has been shown to affect directly the degree to which a surface will cause clots. Clots will form immediately around a positive electrode placed in a blood vessel and will be inhibited by a negative electrode. It has been found that the inner surface of a blood vessel is negatively charged, and that an injury causes it to become positively charged. Sawyer [15] defined a precipitation potential at which red cells were attracted to a positive electrode and found that metals with an oxidation potential higher than the precipitation potential remained clot free for long periods of time.

Following this work many attempts were made to relate Sawyer's findings to the surface charge, or zeta potential, of different materials. The zeta potential is a surface ion effect and does not represent a true net charge. A true electrical charge, such as was used by Sawyer, supports an electric field that can cause ions to move; for example, glass has a highly negative zeta potential but causes rapid clotting. Although there are many exceptions, the evidence indicates that there is no simple relationship between zeta potential and clotting activity.

An approach to reducing clotting that has proven fruitful has been to change the character of the surfaces by either a coating or by chemical alteration; for example, siliconization of glass vessels, which decreases but does not completely prevent clotting, is standard practice in hematological laboratories when unaltered and unclotted blood is needed.

The first nonthrombogenic surface was developed by Gott [17] in 1963. It consisted of a coating of colloidal graphite on a polymeric substrate. The graphite was treated with a benzalkonium chloride and then with heparin, which is one of the most powerful anticoagulants known. The theory of this procedure is that the nonpolar alkyl portion of the benzalkonium ion is adsorbed onto the graphite surface, resulting in a new surface that contains quaternary ammonium groups that are capable of forming a highly nondissociable complex with heparin. Gott describes experiments in which these surfaces remained unclotted for periods of more than a year. Experiments with radioactive heparin showed that significant amounts of heparin remained on the surface (called GBH, for graphite-benzalkonium-heparin) after more than a year. It has been suggested that the heparin supply was actually replenished by heparin carried in the blood. The exact mechanism by which the

Polymer	Clothing Time (min)		Tissue Thromboplastin Times (sec)
	Base Polymer	Heparinized Polymer	
Polystyrene	12		30
Polyethylene	11		—
Silicone rubber	12		45
Polypropylene	12		30
Cellophane	6		—
Vinyl pyridine-butadiene rubber	12		—
Teflon	10	All greater than 60 min	45
Natural rubber	8		30
Epoxy	13		—
Polyvinyl flouride	10		40
Polyvinylidene flouride	12		45
Hydrin rubber	9		45
Ethylene/Propylene rubber	13		—
Styrene butadiene rubber	12		—
Flourinated silicone rubber	8		50
Polyethylene terephtalate film	10		45
Glass	3.5		

Figure 8.9　Properties of some nonthrombogenic polymers. (After Falb.)

GBH surface works is not known. It is interesting that the interiors of blood vessels (the intima) normally contain heparin; the mechanism of action of GBH may prove to be quite physiologic.

The major disadvantage of GBH is that it is brittle and so cannot be used to coat flexible or elastic materials. Some recent approaches to this problem have resulted in a nonthrombogenic cellophane (of great importance for the artificial kidney) by polymerizing ethyleneimine on the surface and then heparinizing it. A mixture of heparin and silicone rubber has also been used successfully for heart valves. The success of GBH started investigations into the possibility of bonding heparin directly to the surface of polymers; this would eliminate the need for a coating and permit developing nonthrombogenic materials that are elastic and flexible. Work at the Battelle Institute in this field has resulted in the development of over 15 nonthrombogenic polymers [14].

Heparin has been attached to the polymers through the incorporation of a quaternary ammonium salt on the surface. Because heparin forms a tight bond with such salts, a surface containing these groups is capable of binding

Polymer	Base Polymer	After Heparinization
Polystyrene	16	50
Polyethylene	25	200
Silicone rubber	5	40
Polypropylene	14	60
Cellophane[a]	600	600
Vinyl pyridine-butadiene rubber	37	75
Teflon	27	8
Natural rubber	13	22
Hydrin rubber	46	69
Ethylene/Propylene rubber	14	65
Styrene butadiene rubber	15	26
Fluorinated silicone rubber	14	33
Glass	3	—

[a] Data on films are doubtful.

FIGURE. 8.10. Hemolytic activity. Hemolysis in mg % hemoglobin. (From Falb, Grode, Luttinger and Leininger.)

heparin. Some of the methods that have been used for preparing these surfaces are as follows:

1. Surface-reaction procedures in which advantage is taken of the chemical reactivity of the functional groups in the polymer.

2. Radiation grafting techniques in which amines such as 4-vinylpyridine are attached or in which a layer of styrene is polymerized on the surface.

3. Use of polymers that contain amine groups in their structure or in cross-linking agents.

4. Inclusion of a polymerizable quaternary ammonium salt into the bulk of the polymer.

The application of these techniques has resulted in over 15 polymers that do not cause clotting in vitro. The results of some of these tests are summarized in Figure 8.9. Figure 8.10 indicates that the heparinized polymers are only slightly more hemolytic than the nonheparinized ones.

2. METALS IN THE BODY

Until relatively recent times the orthopedic surgeons alone worried much about the reactions of metals in the body, because they used metal plates to splint fractured bones. Many of the early implanted devices of the type discussed in this book, such as the pacemaker, avoided the use of metal by encasing as much of the device as possible in plastic. Only platinum was used as an exposed metal because it is almost completely inert in the body. The use of platinum will not be possible however with some of the newer devices, such as the artificial heart, because the amount of metal exposed would make the cost prohibitive. Furthermore, the best way to obtain a good watertight seal is to use metal encapsulation with a welded seam. Offhand, it would seem sufficient to cover the metal with a layer of plastic; therefore the characteristics of the metal would seem to be unimportant. However, since the plastics are permeable to moisture, the layer would have to be very thick to

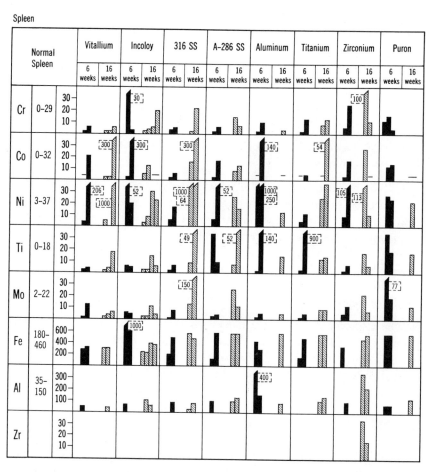

Figure 8.11 Concentrations of trace metals in the spleen. (From [18], used with permission.)

insure that no metal ions could migrate outward. All things considered, it is obviously undesirable to have metals in contact with the tissues.

In attempting to establish the suitability of a particular metal in the body it is necessary to evaluate what happens to metal after implantation and what happens to the surrounding tissues. There is in addition, of course, the important problem of the mechanical suitability of the metal in regard to its tensile strength, flexibility, and fatigue resistance. These aspects are properly in the field of conventional strength of materials and are not discussed here, except as already covered in the section on electrodes.

A thorough study of the fate of implanted metals was made by Ferguson

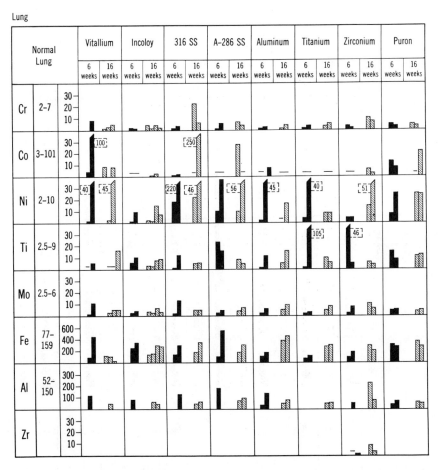

Figure 8.12 Concentrations of metals in the lungs. (From [18], used with permission.)

[18] and his co-workers. In these experiments specimens of commonly used alloys were implanted in rabbits, and subsequently spectrochemical analyses were made of the liver, spleen, kidney, lung, and muscle immediately surrounding and remote from the implant. The metals considered were Vitallium, Incoloy, 316 stainless steel, A–286 stainless steel, aluminum (2024–T3), titanium, zirconium, and Puron. Platinum was used as a control material in this work (some of the surgical instruments were fabricated from it), so no data were presented on this widely used metal.

Metal plugs of the test alloy were embedded in a row in the back muscle of each rabbit, usually six to a rabbit. The surface area of each plug varied between 2.4034 and 3.6948 in.^{2}, and weighed between 16.09 and 28.16

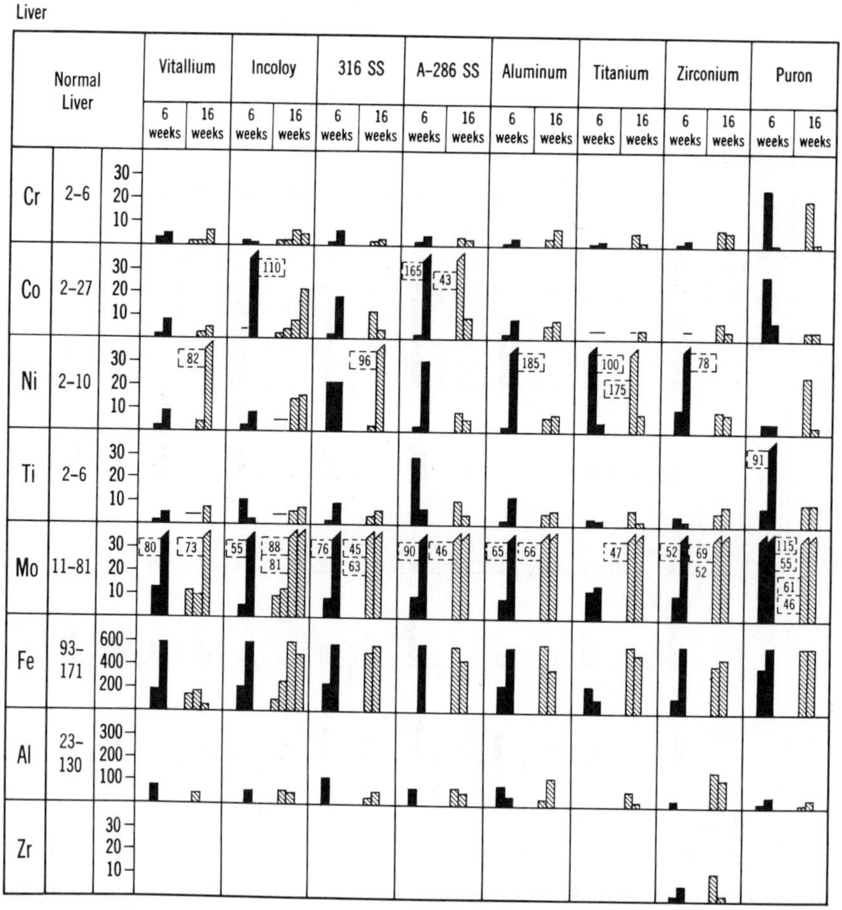

Liver

	Normal Liver		Vitallium		Incoloy		316 SS		A–286 SS		Aluminum		Titanium		Zirconium		Puron	
			6 weeks	16 weeks	6 weeks	16 weeks	6 weeks	16 weeks	6 weeks	16 weeks	6 weeks	16 weeks	6 weeks	16 weeks	6 weeks	16 weeks	6 weeks	16 weeks
Cr	2–6	30 20 10																
Co	2–27	30 20 10			[110]				[165]	[43]								
Ni	2–10	30 20 10	[82]				[96]				[185]		[100] [175]		[78]			
Ti	2–6	30 20 10															[91]	
Mo	11–81	30 20 10	[80]	[73]	[55]	[88] [81]	[76]	[45] [63]	[90]	[46]	[65]	[66]		[47]	[52] [69] 52		[115] [55] [61] [46]	
Fe	93–171	600 400 200																
Al	23–130	300 200 100																
Zr		30 20 10																

Figure 8.13 Concentrations of metals in the liver. (From [18], used with permission.)

grams. Since the rabbits weighed between 1300 and 2700 grams, the weight of the metal was about one-thirtieth to one-fortieth of the body weight. (This would be equivalent to 539 to 1750 grams of the alloy in a 70-kg man.) The plugs were removed over a period of 6 to 16 weeks with glass knives. The results of the study are shown in Figures 8.11 through 8.22. In these figures the results from the same animal are recorded in the same position of each box in the vertical columns, so that the results for a particular animal are in horizontal line. Figures 8.11 through 8.14, which are organized by organ, show the contributions of each implanted alloy to the materials found in the organs. Figures 8.15 through 8.22 show the amounts of the elements

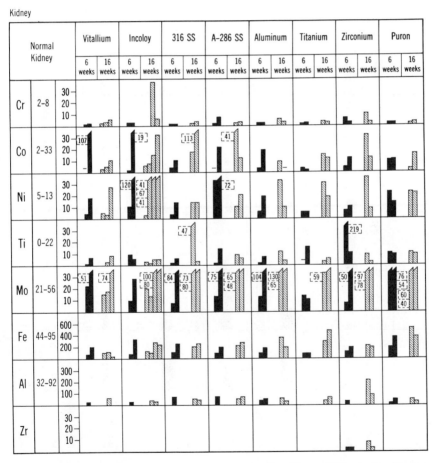

Figure 8.14 Concentrations of metals in the kidneys. (From [18], used with permission.)

chromium, cobalt, nickel, titanium, molybdenum, iron, and aluminum that appeared in the varius organs. The former set of figures can also be used to infer corrosion rates in the body for the various alloys when they are implanted in the body, because the metals found in the body must correspond to the material that has corroded from the implant, exclusive of components that have been excreted.

The concentrations of trace ions are recorded as parts per million of dry

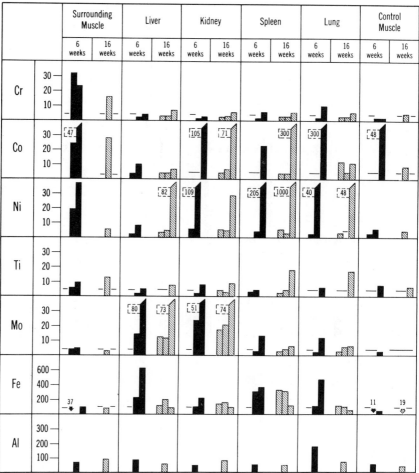

Figure 8.15   Concentration of Vitallium in various organs. (From [18], used with permission.)

ash. Each figure of the last eight gives, at the top, the results for one implant whose concentration is shown in the figures in parentheses. Each bar is the mean of two determinations from one animal. To save space high values are indicated by bars with slanting tops, with the figure in the adjacent flag giving the actual numerical results. Horizontal lines indicate that no ion was found, and results too small to be represented by a bar are indicated by arrows with the actual numerical values.

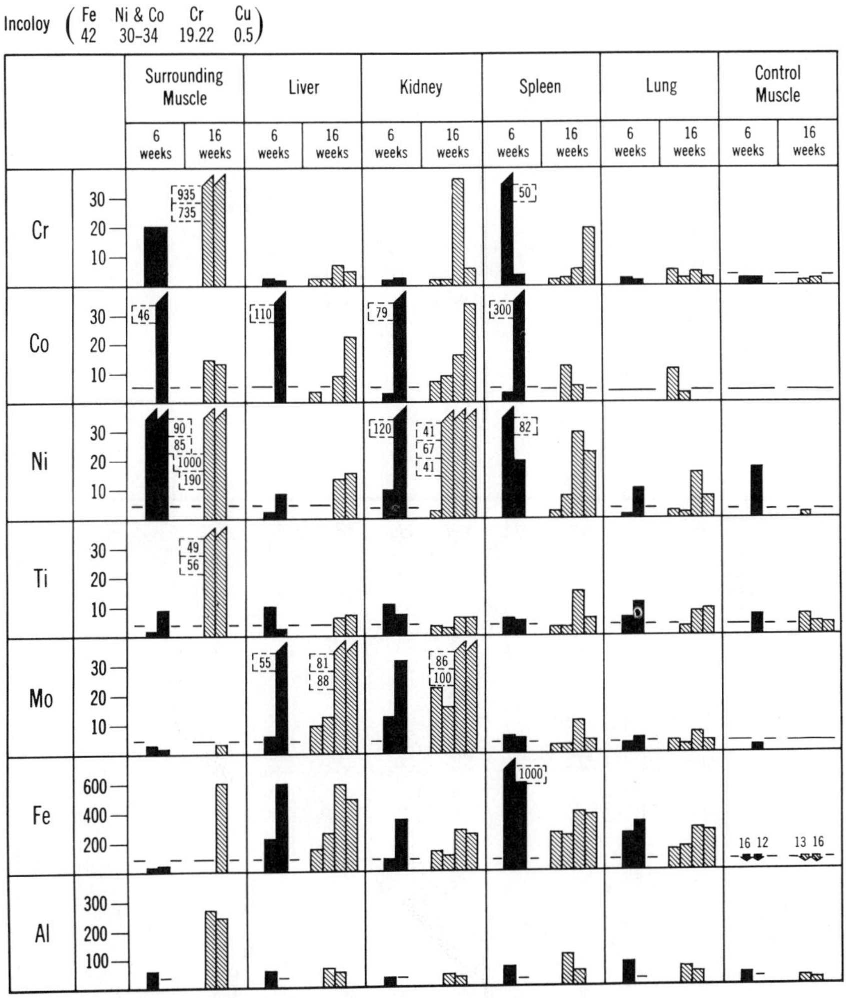

Figure 8.16 Concentration of Incoloy in various organs. (From [18], used with permission.)

Some general patterns are apparent in these results. Perhaps the most surprising result is that metals that are often thought of as being quite inert distribute themselves so widely over the body. Stainless steel contributed nickel to the body circulation, and cobalt-based materials contributed cobalt. Iron enters prominently into normal metabolism, so any iron contributed by the implants probably has a negligible effect; the only widespread change was noted with almost pure iron in the form of Puron. If an experimental ani-

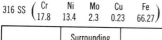

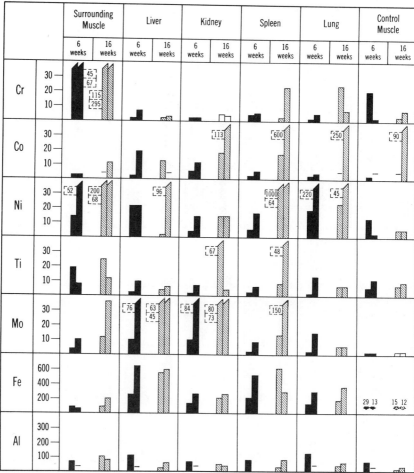

Figure 8.17   Concentration of A-286 stainless steel in organs. (From [18], used with permission.)

mal showed an unusual tendency to pick up one type of ion, it also tended to pick up other ions. This suggests either accelerated corrosion of the implant or a predisposition of the animal to use and store the particular metals. It is also conceivable that differences between the animals contributed to different corrosion rates. If individual differences are significant, then this must be determined before making an implant of a prosthetic device.

The spleen and lung led the list in the storage of trace metals, with the

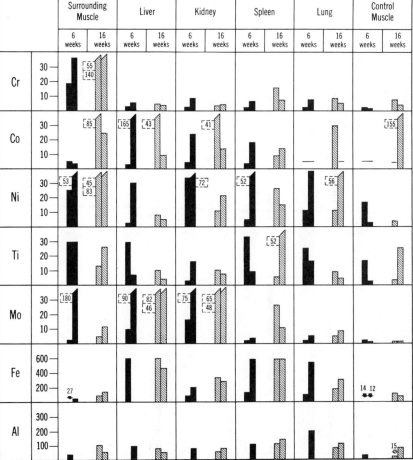

Figure 8.18 Concentration of 316 stainless steel in organs. (From [18], used with permission.)

liver and kidney second. The muscle surrounding the implant always had a significant concentration of the metal, but control muscle from elsewhere in the body did not pick up the metal. The spleen appeared to be able to store chromium, cobalt, titanium, nickel, iron, aluminum, and zirconium, but it was not determined whether these materials were merely held in the organ or whether they entered actively into the metabolism. By contrast, relatively small increases in trace-metal concentrations were found in the liver. The

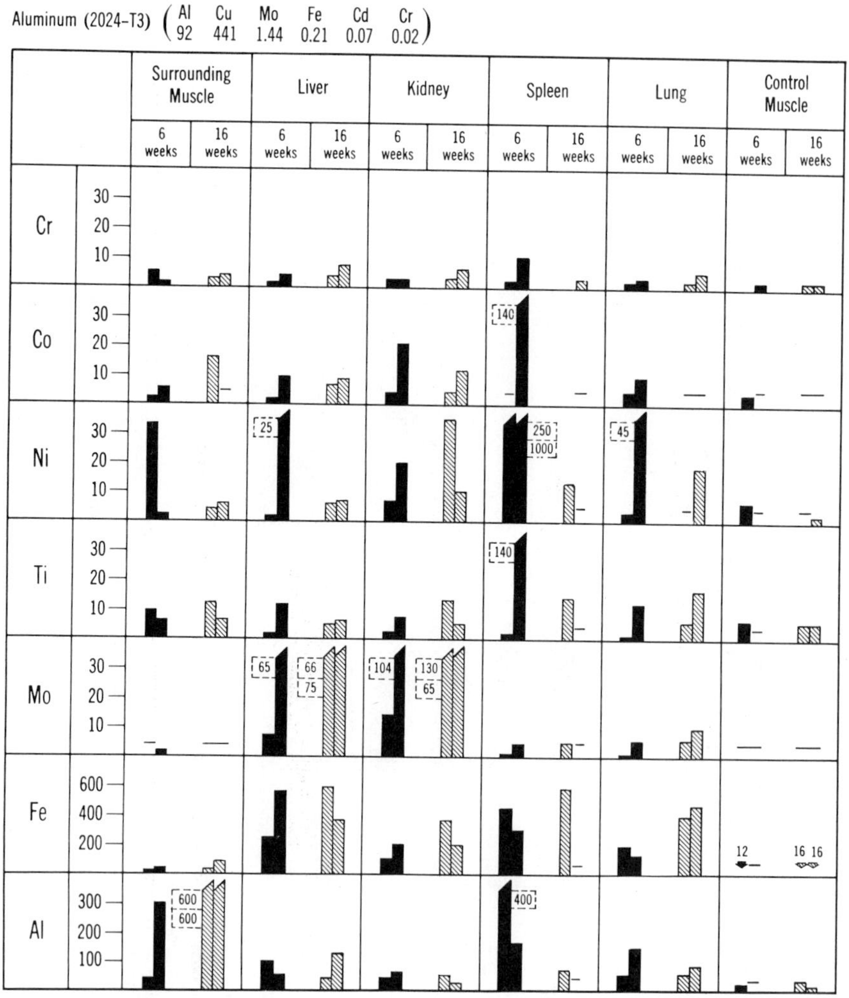

Aluminum (2024–T3) $\left(\begin{array}{cccccc} Al & Cu & Mo & Fe & Cd & Cr \\ 92 & 441 & 1.44 & 0.21 & 0.07 & 0.02 \end{array}\right)$

Figure 8.19   Concentration of Aluminum in organs. (From [18], used with permission.)

lung had particularly high levels of cobalt and nickel but not of other materials. The kidney also tended to retain cobalt and nickel.

The concentration of iron in all of the organs analyzed was raised slightly by most implanted alloys, even those that did not contain much iron.

Cobalt and nickel were found more frequently than chromium, but the molybdenum concentration was not appreciably increased by any of the im-

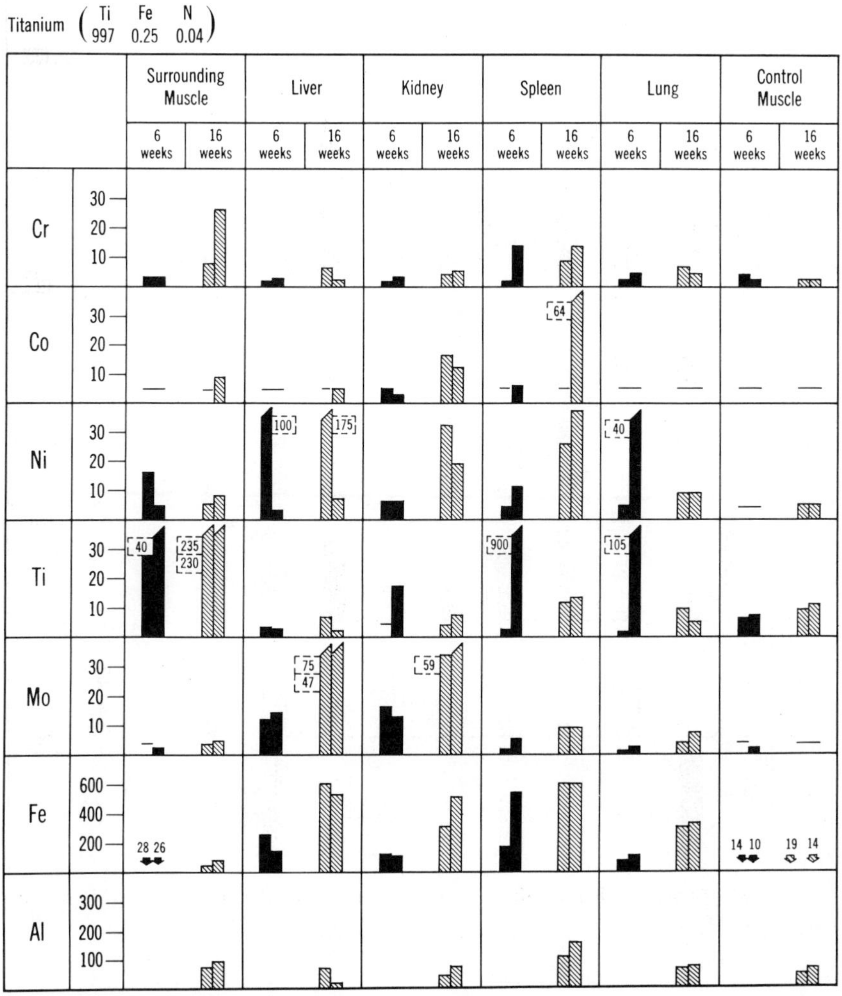

Figure 8.20 Concentration of Titanium in organs. (From [18], used with permission.)

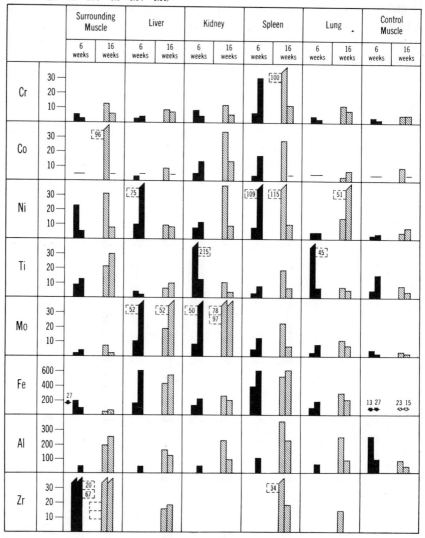

Figure 8.21 Concentration of Zirconium in organs. (From [18], used with permission.)

plants. Titanium and zirconium were readily stored in all organs at low levels.

Only the more active alloys and ions showed changes in the tissue levels of trace elements between 6 and 16 weeks. In the spleen all elements, with the exception of iron, tended to increase with time. In the lung the general trend was to clear trace elements from the tissue, except for the cobalt from the 316 stainless steel. The liver showed only small differences between 6 and 16 weeks; apparently trace ions were eliminated, except for titanium. The kidneys showed only a reduction of the trace materials.

Puron (Fe 99)

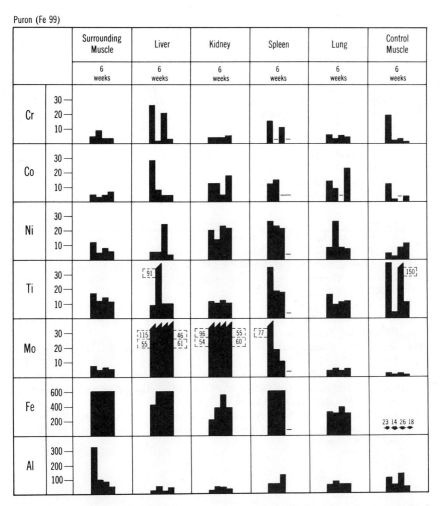

Figure 8.22 Concentration of Puron in organs. (From [18], used with permission.)

Thus the spleen was the one organ that tended to increase trace-metal concentration with time.

REFERENCES

[1] Braley, S., "The Medical Silicones," *Trans. ASAIO,* X:240 (1964).

[2] American Society for Testing Materials, *Plastics in Surgical Implants,* ASTM Special Publication No. 386, 1965.

[3] Folkman, J., and D. Long, "Drug Pacemakers in the Treatment of Heart Block," *Ann. N. Y. Acad. Sci.,* III:848 (Art. 3), June 1964.

[4] Davila, J. C., "Development of Artificial Heart Valves," *Plastics in Surgical Implants,* ASTM Special Publication No. 386, 1965, p. 1.

[5] Leininger, R. I., "Changes in Properties of Plastics during Implantations," ibid., p. 71.

[6] Harrison, reported by Leininger in [5].

[7] Turner, F., reported by S. Woodward in "Biological End Points for Compatibility," *Plastics in Surgery Implants,* op. cit., p. 77.

[8] Oppenheimer, B., reported by Woodward, ibid.

[9] Alexander, P., and E. Horning, reported by Woodward, ibid.

[10] Woodward, S., ibid.

[11] Sears, David, "Effects of Implants on the Blood," *Plastics in Surgery Implants,* op. cit., p. 88.

[12] Shea, M., R. Indeglia, F. Dorman, J. Halein, P. Blackshear, L. Varco, and E. Bernstein, "The Biologic Response to Pumping Blood," *Trans. ASAIO,* XIII:116 (1967).

[13] Sawyer, P., S. Srinivasan, S. Wesolowski, K. Berger, A. Campbell, A. Sammar, S. Wood, and L. Sauvage, "Development and in Vivo Evaluation of Metals for Heart Valve Prosthesis," *Trans. ASAIO,* XIII:131 (1967).

[14] This discussion is based on Falb, R., G. A. Grode, M. L. Luttinger, and R. I. Leininger, "Polymeric Materials in Bioengineering," *Proc. Ann. Conf. on Eng. in Med. and Biol.,* 8:261 (1966).

[15] Harshein, D., H. Ziskind, S. Wesolowski, and P. Sawyer, "The Ionic Structure of the Blood Intimal Interface as an Aid in the Development of Vascular Prostheses," *Trans. ASAIO,* IX:317 (1963).

[16] Lyman, D., "Biomedical Polymers," *Ann. N. Y. Acad. Sci.,* 146:30 (Art. 1) (1968).

[17] Gott, V., J. Whiffen, D. Koepke, R. Dagget, W. Booke, and W. Young, "Techniques of Applying a Graphite-Benzalkonium-Heparin Coating to Various Plastics and Metals," *Trans. ASAIO,* X:213 (1964).

[18] Ferguson, A. B., Jr., Y. Akahoshi, P. Laing, and E. Hodge, "Characteristics of Trace Ions Released from Embedded Metal," *J. Bone and Joint Surgery,* 44A:32, March 1962.

CHAPTER NINE

The Heart as a Pump

In preceding chapters the mechanism by which the heart rate is controlled has been discussed. This led quite naturally into a discussion of the cardiac pacemaker, which is used as an artificial organ when the heart's own pacemaker cannot regulate the heartbeat properly; and the carotid-sinus pacemaker, which acts as a replacement for the basic sensor that regulates the blood pressure. In this section the heart as a mechanical pump is considered. The natural heart is discussed first, followed by a description of some of the better known heart substitutes and mechanisms for their fabrication.

The heart is a simple two-stroke pump (actually a pair of pumps) with automatic valves, very similar in its basic operation to the small bilge pump used in small boats; but the heart, of course, is not a piston pump. The two "strokes" are the filling phase and the emptying, or power, phase. As in the bilge pump, the valve action is purely passive: whenever the pressure on one side of the valve is greater than on the other, the valve automatically opens or closes.

The two sides of the heart, left and right, act quite independently, mechanically, and the efficiency of the heart does not depend on their being synchronous. The contractions are approximately synchronous, only because the two pumps have a common pacemaker and a parallel system of Purkinje fibers. Events following the stimulations caused by the pacemaker are completely independent in the two ventricles, although as a matter of fact they almost coincide in time.

The basic flow of blood through the heart can be visualized with the help of Figure 9.1. The heart is divided into four chambers, the left and right atria [1, 2], and the left and right ventricles. Oxygen-poor blood enters the right atrium from the superior and inferior vena cava. The blood then passes into the right ventricle, where it is ejected into the pulmonary circulation by way of the pulmonary artery and becomes oxygenated. It returns by way of the pulmonary veins to the left atrium, then goes into the left ventricle, where it is pumped to the rest of the body through the aorta. The left atrium, ventricle, aorta, and branches are known as the *systemic* circulation—in contrast

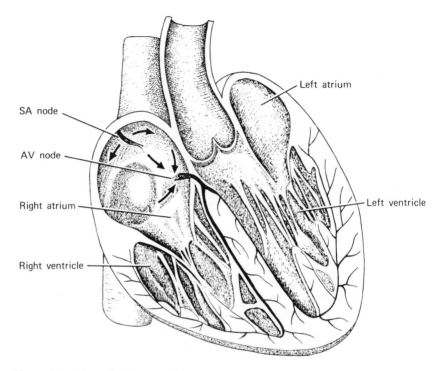

Figure 9.1   Schematic diagram of heart.

to the *pulmonary* circulation, which is the circuit of the right atrium, ventricle, and lungs, where oxygenation occurs.

There are many confusing definitions of the words "systole" and "diastole." The words originally described the period when the heart was pumping as contrasted to the period when it was filling—or *activity* versus *rest*. As can be seen from the brief discussion just presented, as well as the description of the electrical activity of the heart, mechanical ventricular systole is different from mechanical aortic systole, and they are all different from the electrical systole and diastole. It is generally agreed, however, that *systolic pressure* is the maximum arterial pressure during a pulse, and *diastolic pressure* is the lowest pressure reached. Although it is possible to split hairs over just what events are to be included under each, it is really not worthwhile to make the definitions any more precise.

The contraction of the atria plays only a minor role in pumping, although it assists in the filling of the ventricles. For the atrium to pump to any significant degree there would have to be valves upstream from the atria to prevent reflux of blood into the systemic circuit or lungs. (Such a valve is actually found in the single-chambered heart of the fish.) In describing the heart as a pump, therefore, the action of the ventricles will be concentrated on. This statement should not be taken to imply that the atria may be dispensed with: some investigators designing artificial hearts found that they could not be made to work properly without providing the reservoir of blood in the atria.

The sequence of contraction of the ventricles from apex to base has been described as a milking action. It is interesting to note that when the heart beats about as much blood remains behind in the ventricles (70 ml on the average) as is ejected (80 ml). The efficiency of the heart is not related to whether it empties completely: the blood remaining in the ventricles provides a variable reservoir of blood that can be utilized in varying the stroke volume.

Although the heart cycle can be subdivided into many phases, four basic ones are sufficient to understand its operation. These are based on combinations of inlet valve open or closed, and of outlet valve open or closed. The combination of inlet and outlet valves both open does not occur in the normal heart with good valves. The four are:

1. Filling (inlet open, outlet closed);
2. Isovolumetric contraction (inlet closed, outlet closed);
3. Ejection (inlet closed, outlet open);
4. Isovolumetric relaxation (inlet closed, outlet closed).

These phases are shown schematically in Figure 9.2, together with graphs of cardiac volume, and ventricular and aortic pressure.

1. *Filling.* In ventricular diastole, when the ventricles relax, the pressure in the ventricle falls to only a few millimeters of mercury. The atrioventricular valves open when the ventricular pressure drops below the atrial pressure, and blood flows into the ventricle. The ventricular muscle relaxes still more, so that the ventricular pressure continues to fall for a short time and filling becomes rapid, a period lasting approximately 0.1 sec. After this the rate of filling diminishes because the ventricular pressure rises slightly when the chamber becomes full. During all of this filling phase the inlet valves (the mitral or the tricuspid valve) of the ventricle all open. The outlet valves (aortic or pulmonary) are closed because the pressure in the aorta and the pulmonary artery is much higher than it is in the ventricles.

The filling phase ends when the initial contraction of the ventricular muscle raises the ventricular pressure above the atrial pressure, at which time the atrioventricular valves close. The total filling period lasts for more than half of the cardiac cycle at normal heart rates, but less when the rate is increased.

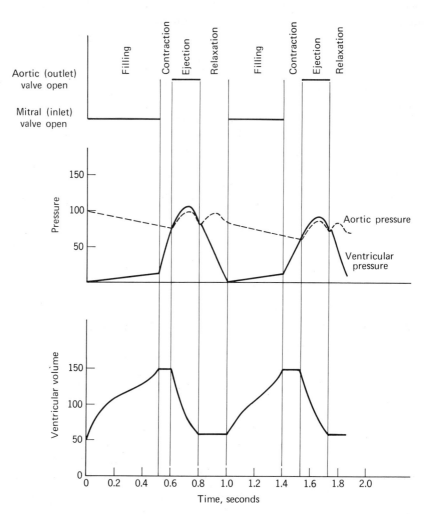

Figure 9.2 Pressure and volume changes in the heart correlated with various valve openings and closures. (After Burton.)

2. Isovolumetric Contraction. The ventricle is now a closed space because both valves are shut and there can be no change in ventricular volume, although the shape changes as the wall develops tension. The ventricle becomes more spherical, and as the contraction develops more tension in the wall the pressure within the chamber rises rapidly. When it exceeds the pressure remaining in the aorta (which in the meantime has been dropping by runoff from the last beat) the outlet valves (aortic or pulmonary valve) open, ending the phase.

3. *Ejection.* The blood in the ventricle is now ejected into the aorta at a rate faster than the blood in the aorta can empty into the tissues. The pressure in the aorta thus rises with that in the ventricle (because they have in effect become a common chamber) and continues to rise during contraction.

Between one-half and two-thirds of the way through the ejection phase the contraction of the ventricle stops and it relaxes rapidly. The ventricular pressure falls because of the relaxation; but, since it falls more slowly than the aortic pressure can fall by runoff, ejection continues. However, ventricular relaxation becomes faster while aortic runoff decreases, so the ventricular pressure soon falls below the aortic pressure and the aortic valve snaps shut, ending the ejection phase. It lasts about 0.2 sec at normal heart rates. Its end is marked by a notch on the aortic pressure curve (the dicrotic notch).

4. *Isovolumetric Relaxation.* The ventricle is again a closed chamber in which the volume cannot change (although the shape does). The pressure falls rapidly as the tension in the ventricular muscle decreases. The pressure eventually falls to below the atrial pressure, causing the opening of the atrioventricular valve and ending the phase in less than 0.1 sec.

As mentioned before, the inlet and outlet valves are never open at the same time. If they were, pumping would be inefficient. In disease distortion of the valve leaflets causes incompetence (sometimes called insufficiency) of the valves so that blood can still return through them when they are closed. Aortic incompetence causes *aortic regurgitation.* After the aortic valve has closed blood will flow back into the relaxing heart because the aortic pressure exceeds the ventricular pressure, which wastes much of the heart's work. A similar situation can occur with the pulmonary valve. Incompetence of the inlet valves (mitral and tricuspid) leads to backflow into the atria.

The blood circuit from the vena cava, through the right ventricle, pulmonary arteries, lungs, and pulmonary veins is called the pulmonary circulation (or circulation through the *right side* of the heart). The circuit through the left ventricle, aorta, major arteries, capillaries of organs, veins, and vena cava, is the systemic system, or circulation of the *left side* of the heart. It is sometimes clearer to use such simple designations in descriptions of the circulatory systems.

The function of the heart is to force blood through the blood vessels and eventually to supply oxygen to the tissues by way of the capillaries. There are a large number of parallel routes by which blood can pass from the high-pressure side of the arterial circulation to the low-pressure side of the veins. Since these paths are in parallel, the flow through each of them is not affected

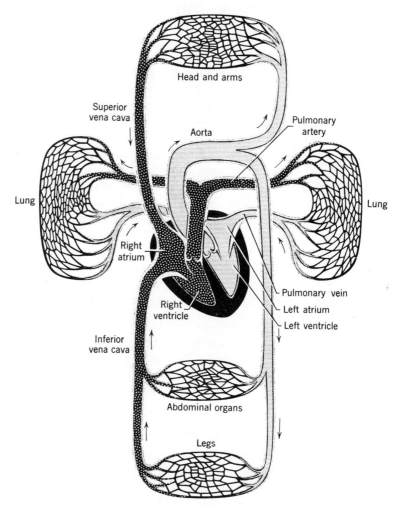

Figure 9.3   Schematic diagram showing various routes of the circulation.

directly by the others but depends only on the driving pressure. The thousands of paths can be divided into several categories, as shown in Figure 9.3.

1. Simple routes in which a single bed of capillaries is supplied in each route. Most routes are of this type, including the circulation of the head and limbs, the coronary circulation, and the liver.

2. Routes in which two sets of capillaries are arranged in series; for example, the kidneys.

3. Routes in which more than two sets of capillaries are supplied. This is

FIGURE 9.4 Geometry of Mesenteric Vascular Bed of the Dog[a]

	Aorta	Large arteries	Main artery branches	Terminal branches	Acterioles	Capillaries	Venules	Terminal veins	Main venous branches	Large veins	Vena cave
Diameter (mm)	10	3	1	0.6	0.02	0.008	0.03	1.5	2.4	6.0	12.5
Number in category	1	40	6×10^2	1.8×10^3	4×10^7	1.2×10^9	8×10^7	1.8×10^3	6×10^2	40	1
Total Cross-Sectional area (cm²)	0.8	3.0	5.0	25	125	600	570	30	27	11	1.2
Total Volume (cm³)	30	60	50	25	25	60	110	30	270	220	50

[a] Data from reference 1.

133

true of the portal system (the system draining the intestines) in which the capillaries of the spleen are in parallel with those of the intestine, and both are in series with the capillaries of the liver.

4. The pulmonary circulation, which is unique because it is a path from the high-pressure right side of the heart to the low-pressure left side of the heart instead of being a path from the aorta to the vena cava.

5. The bronchial circulation, which is also unique. It is the minor system supplying the lung tissue itself and acts as a shunt across the left heart only, returning blood to the left atrium without ever passing through the lung air spaces to become oxygenated.

Another difference is the location of control points. These are vessels whose constriction can control the flow of blood through the vascular beds and are known as arterioles (or resistance vessels). In the first category there is a single set of control points before the single capillary bed, whereas in the second and third categories there are multiple sets.

Each of these main routes has many elements in series, and each element has many similar vessels in parallel. The blood travels from a main artery through many parallel distributing arteries and arterioles to the capillaries. It then converges into venules, then collecting veins, to a main vein, and finally empties into the vena cava. The geometry of this system in the dog is shown in Figure 9.4. It is generally believed that these figures are typical of vascular beds in general. The data show that every time there is a branching into a larger total number of vessels in parallel the total cross-sectional area increases until at the level of the capillaries it is 800 times that of the aorta. After that the vessels converge, and the cross-sectional area decreases. The area of the vena cava is only 50 percent greater than that of the aorta.

The method by which the heart regulates its output is of great importance in designing an artificial replacement. The basic problem arises because the heart is actually two pumps in series, as is illustrated in Figure 9.5. Suppose (as is shown in the figure) that there were two pumps whose outputs could be adjusted to some chosen value but were not automatically controlled. The pumps are shown in series with two "vascular systems," which are supposed to correspond to the pulmonary and systemic circulations. In general it would be impossible without some sort of servomechanism to make the outputs of the two hearts identical. Suppose that one pump had an output of 5.0 liters/ min, whereas the other, due to errors in setting it, had an output of 5.1 liters/ min. Then 0.1 liters of fluid would be carried every minute from one circulation to the other. The blood volume is normally divided so that about 3.3 liters is in the systemic part and 1.7 liters in the pulmonary. In 10 minutes, in this hypothetical example, 1 liter of blood would be transferred from one

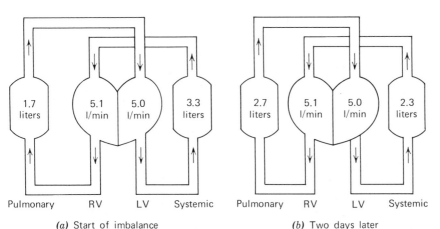

Pulmonary   RV   LV   Systemic   Pulmonary   RV   LV   Systemic

(*a*) Start of imbalance   (*b*) Two days later

Figure 9.5 Schematic diagram showing effects of imbalance in left and right heart: (*a*) start of imbalance; (*b*) two days later. (After Burton.)

circulation to the other. This would create a situation incompatible with life.

It is necessary therefore to have some automatic method of maintaining the volumes in the two circulatory systems constant. One method by which this is accomplished in the normal heart is stated by Starling's law, that "the energy of contraction of the ventricular muscle is a function of the length of the muscle fiber"; for example, if the ventricles are filled to a greater extent, the following systolic contraction is more forceful, and a greater stroke volume is ejected. By this mechanism in any time period the outputs of the left and

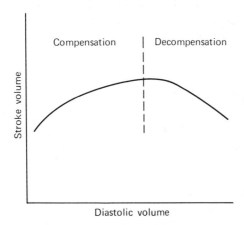

Figure 9.6 Schematic diagram illustrating Starling's law.

right ventricles are approximately equal, and the total blood volume remains distributed in the proper proportions between the systemic and pulmonary circulations.

The experimental basis for the law is illustrated in Figure 9.6. At first the stroke volume increases with the diastolic volume. After the heart is filled to a critical point further increase in volume leads to a decrease in stroke volume. This is called the *decompensation* stage. This curve probably depends on the fact that the strength of contraction of a cardiac fiber increases, up to a point, as the initial length of tension increases. There is very little direct experimental evidence performed on isolated muscle fibers of this last property because of the difficulty of obtaining the isolated fiber.

It is now possible to see how Starling's law maintains the proper cardiac output. The outputs of the two hearts are seldom identical during any single beat. As a matter of fact, during expiration the output of the right heart is considerably greater than the output of the left heart. However, this increased output of the right heart increases the filling of the left heart a few beats later, and by Starling's law its output increases correspondingly, preventing any accumulation in the pulmonary circulation.

Another method often used to maintain volume distribution with two pumps in series is to use a "bleeder," or shunt, across one of the pumps. If a progressive shift of volume into one of the circulations occurred, the mean pressure there would rise and the flow through the shunt would then change in order to compensate. Such a procedure would prevent large shifts of fluid but would not regulate the pressures and volumes within very narrow limits. In fact the circulatory system has such a shunt provided by the bronchial circulation, which is a path from the aorta to the pulmonary veins and left atrium, in effect a shunt across the left side of the heart. It is not known how important this path is in regulating blood flow. In cases where the automatic control by Starling's law does not operate because of diseased heart muscle it may become quite important.

REFERENCES

[1] Burton, A. C., *Physiology and Biophysics of the Circulation,* Year Book Medical Publishers, Chicago, 1965.
[2] Rushmer, R., *Cardiovascular Dynamics,* Saunders, Philadelphia, 1961.

CHAPTER TEN

Artificial Hearts and Assisted Circulation

The preceding chapter presented a brief outline of the physiology of the normal heart, including its pumping and regulatory mechanisms. This section presents some of the technical work being done on artificial hearts and various types of heart substitutes. A preliminary discussion of the physiology of the artificial heart (as contrasted with that of the natural heart) is followed by a discussion of the types of pumps actually used and some of the engineering problems that are met in their design and use. The materials problems, insofar as they affect the biological applications of the devices, are mainly covered in the appropriate chapters. The section concludes with a discussion of how the pumps have actually been applied in various cases.

Two distinct aspects of cardiac support are discussed here. The first, which is most properly known as the artificial heart, is a total replacement for either the entire heart or a portion of it (usually one or both ventricles). The second aspect, which has more immediate application, is assisted circulation, or AC. This refers to booster pumps for the natural heart for limited periods of time. In many cases of acute heart failure a temporary aid to the heart permits the body's healing processes to repair any damage that has occurred, and an additional pump, either in series or in parallel with the subject's own heart, can take an appreciable amount of the pumping load for restricted periods of time (a few hours to several days). The heart-lung machine used during open chest surgical procedures is in a somewhat intermediate state. It is a total replacement for the heart but is used only for short periods of time (typically several hours). The question naturally arises as to the definition of "heart failure," and the conditions under which these devices should be used are of considerable importance. Following Salisbury [1], heart failure will be somewhat arbitrarily defined as a condition characterized by at least one of the following:

1. Abnormally high diastolic pressure in the failing ventricle;

2. Excessive pulmonary (or systemic) venous pressure when the cardiac output is adequate (above about 50 ml/kg-min);

3. Existence of "vicious circles" that cause progressive circulatory and chemical deterioration, and finally death.

Physicians and surgeons have treated such cases by varying methods for many years, so the question naturally arises as to when assisted circulation should be used. Those who advocate this method of treatment should consider it when self-perpetuating abnormalities exist; for example, decreased cardiac output caused by the failing heart can reduce the circulation to the heart itself so that a vicious circle is set up, and the subject's condition continually worsens. Similarly, insufficient output can cause chemical changes (such as acidosis) that tend to perpetuate themselves. When heart failure has reached an irreversible point as yet not clearly defined, assisted circulation or total replacement may be the only effective treatment. At this writing only assisted circulation has been attempted clinically with artificial devices, although natural replacements have been attempted.

At the present state of the art acute heart failure seems to offer the widest field of application for assisted circulation. Intuitively it is felt that "tired" hearts need "rest," which can be supplied by having part of its work taken over by an auxiliary pump. This intuitive feeling has scientific support in data that indicate that assisted circulation may break self-perpetuating vicious circles that intensify heart failure and eventually cause death.

There are two principal intrinsic conditions of the cardiac muscle, either of which is sufficient to bring about the failure of a ventricle: decreased contractile strength, or decreased contractility (weakness); or decreased compliance (excessive stiffness).

The discussion in Chapter 9 concerning Starling's law and the method by which cardiac output is regulated should make it clear why insufficient contractility can cause heart failure. From the explanation given there, it can be seen that the whole mechanism breaks down if there is insufficient force to expel the blood.

Starling's law, when combined with Laplace's law, indicates clearly some of the mechanisms that occur. Laplace's law states that the developed pressure P is proportional to the tension in the wall, T, and inversely proportional to the radius of the vessel, R; thus $P = kT/R$, where k is a constant. If the ventricle becomes overdistended, so that R increases, then the pressure P will decrease for a given tension, resulting in decreased cardiac output. This same phenomenon can be used to explain the decompensation portion of the characteristic of heart muscle already considered under the discussion of Starling's law.

The heart muscle, or *myocardium,* can be weakened in many different ways, some of which are not too well known. Some of the known causes are inadequate pressure in the coronary arteries, insufficient blood flow in the coronary arteries, inadequate oxygen in the arteries, increased acidity of the blood (acidemia, or acidosis), improper levels of various salts in the blood and tissue fluids (electrolyte imbalance), and abnormalities of the mechanism by which the heart is excited. There seem to be many unknown factors that cause disease even when the above factors are not present.

In the second cause of heart failure (i.e., increased stiffness) the ventricle is unable to fill properly, although it can eject and it can produce sufficient contractile tension. This condition coexists with, and is probably caused by, excess fluid (edema) of the heart muscle [1]. Fluid accumulation above the normal water content of the cardiac muscle (77 to 78 percent) is a nonspecific response to almost any kind of myocardial injury. It can also be initiated by the first cause above, since weakness of the heart muscle leads to excessive filling pressure, which can cause edema by forcing the fluid into the tissue.

Heart failure can also occur when the heart has not been injured and can function normally; for example, body temperatures that are lower than normal (hypothermia) can lengthen the systolic phase of the cardiac cycle so much that the filling of the ventricles during diastole is interfered with. Very high heart rates can have a similar effect. Various types of circulatory failure, or shock, include heart failure when there is either low or high cardiac output.

The effects of heart failure are serious even when death does not occur immediately. When either heart failure or circulatory failure has existed for some time the performance of many of the body organs (including the lungs, the nervous system, and endocrine glands) and other parts of the body are modified. These in turn influence the heart and blood vessels in such a way as to magnify the effects that originally caused them, thus creating a vicious circle, or a kind of positive feedback, which ultimately causes death. Only a few of these mechanisms are known; for example, a relatively simple case can be started by left heart failure. If the failure is severe enough to cause fluid in the lungs (pulmonary edema) and interfere with the oxygenation of the blood there (and it is not counteracted by discharge of epinephrine), the underoxygenated arterial blood may cause chemoreceptors to lower the heart rate and overload the heart each beat. At the same time carbon dioxide pressure in the blood rises, blood pH falls, and the contractile strength of the heart muscle is reduced by the acidity of the blood. The low arterial blood oxygen also causes myocardial edema. Thus the original pulmonary edema has weakened the heart, and the deteriorating heart has intensified the pulmonary edema.

There are other cases in which the mechanisms of the positive feedback action are not so obvious. The interdependence of the reflexes that control the size of the blood vessels (vasomotor reflexes), the receptors for which are located in the lungs, the wall of the left ventricle, and carotid arteries and aortic regions is likely to have harmful effects. Changes of the levels of various hormones in the blood can act in a similar way. Deleterious mechanisms occur as a result of damage to the right side of the heart; for example, the dependence of right ventricular contractile strength on coronary pressure has been known since 1888.

A measure of negative feedback is supplied by the mechanism of Starling's law. Usually the output of one side of the heart tends to be reduced in heart failure because the tissue damage is not symmetrically located. As a result that ventricle fills more completely. Starling's law provides a compensatory increase in stroke volume as the diastolic volume increases, thus acting as a negative feedback mechanism. This corrective action can only occur up to the point where decompensation sets in, which is where the dilation exceeds the critical value. The automatic adjustment now becomes a positive feedback mechanism, and the stroke volume decreases with increased dilation, resulting in rapid pulmonary congestion.

From this discussion it can be seen that there are many occasions when assisted circulation would be useful as a temporary method of overcoming transient, but potentially lethal, situations. The frequency of these circumstances provides much of the impetus for the development of assisted-circulation devices. Although total replacements of the heart are important, assisted-circulation devices that could function for several weeks would be of significant importance in reducing mortality.

Of course, there are situations in which assisted circulation is definitely contraindicated; for example, it has been shown that increasing the central coronary pressure may actually damage a failing heart [1]. Such high pressure may stiffen the heart muscle, thereby initiating or intensifying the positive feedback mechanisms already discussed. The precise usefulness of assisted circulation is a matter for medical judgement, and the nature of problems calling for a form of circulatory aid are of some importance in the proper design of the equipment.

There are two basic parts of an artificial heart. The first is the pump, which replaces the basic heart and is the device most people think of as the prosthetic device. The lungs, however, are a component of the cardiac function. It is possible to think of the heart and lungs as a basic element in the body that both oxygenates blood and provides the motive force that makes it circulate. Whereas most of the experimental implantable hearts simply replace the pumping function, most of those currently in use for short-term assistance during open heart operations also oxygenate the blood and therefore are really heart-lung machines (as many of them are actually called). The basic method

Blood in

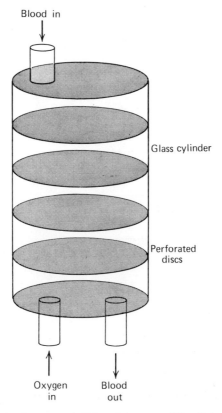

Glass cylinder

Perforated
discs

Oxygen
in

Blood
out

Figure 10.1   Schematic diagram of disk oxygenator. (The disks may also stand on
edge, and rotate through the blood over a central axle.)

by which these oxygenators work is to provide a large surface area for ex-
posure of the blood to an atmosphere in which oxygen and carbon dioxide will
be exchanged according to their relative partial pressures. The principles behind two typical devices are shown schematically in Figures 10.1 and 10.2.
In the device of Figure 10.1 a column contains a large number of perforated
disks through which the blood drips and pressurized oxygen is forced through
the column in the opposite direction. In another common device, shown in
Figure 10.2, the blood passes through a plastic tube filled with a metal sponge
that effectively increases the path length through which the blood must travel
and provides a large surface area for mixing of the blood with the pressurized
oxygen. Unfortunately, none of these devices is satisfactory for prolonged oxygenation because of the damage they cause the blood, mainly by denaturing
the proteins in the blood cells. As a result almost all current designs for im-

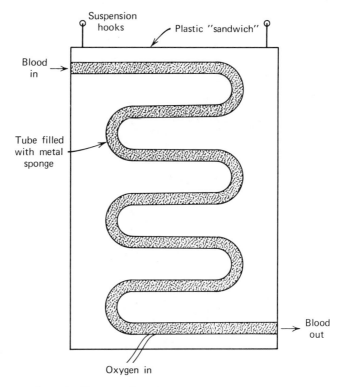

Figure 10.2   Schematic diagram of another type of oxygenator.

plantable hearts are for a pump alone and do not make any provision for any pulmonary functions.

Pumping blood for more than a few hours can cause deleterious physiological effects, and this is one of the major problems that must be solved in the development of an artificial heart. Some of these effects are caused by the typical reactions to foreign bodies in the blood stream, as discussed in the chapter on materials in the body. Some, however, are a direct result of the stresses caused by the mechanical action of the pump. The main problems here are destruction of red blood cells (hemolysis) and clotting (thrombosis). (The means that have been taken to reduce these effects are included under the discussions of the individual types of pumps that have been tested; whereas the allowable levels of these effects, as far as they are known, are covered in the materials chapter, because the problems that must be solved, from an engineering standpoint, are very similar.) One problem that is still under active consideration, however, is whether the flow must be pulsatile, as it is in the normal individual, or whether a continuous steady flow can be used. Almost all of the heart pumps used for short-term operations produce either a continuous flow or else a sinusoidal pulse that is completely different from the pressure wave produced by the normal heart. Many physiologists have attempted to determine just what function the pulsatile flow plays in normal physiology. Some parts of the body, for example, can continue to function with virtually no pulsation in the blood flow, but the effect of absolutely no pulsation has not been tested [2, 3]. During the short periods of external assisted circulation of open heart operations, when the pulsatile flow has the "smooth" characteristics just mentioned, there has been no effect on eventual recovery, but there is no real information concerning what would happen if this situation were maintained indefinitely. The problem has considerable technical importance in designing an artificial heart, because most pumps that create a pulsatile flow are of the reciprocating-positive-displacement type and must have valves at both the input and output parts, with the accompanying hemolysis caused by the mechanical stress of the valves. If pulseless flow were satisfactory, then rotary or centrifugal pumps could be used, some of which have only one moving part. Such pumps would probably be rugged and simple to construct. One of the more complete studies designed to answer this question performed by Rainer [3] showed that the response of a group of dogs subjected to pulsatile flow "reflected a more nearly physiologic state than that of a similar group of animals that received perfusions under 'mean pressure' flow." However, he points out that studies at the microcirculation level are of great importance, since the basic purpose of the circulatory system is to deliver oxygen to the cells. He quotes others who have shown deterioration in arteriolar circulation and the blood vessel wall as a result of nonpulsatile flow, effects that were reversed when the flow was made pulsatile. Also, as might be expected on intuitive grounds, pulsatile flow was better tolerated over long time periods. It may be more for the last reason than for any other that the developers of artificial hearts designed for implantation have tried to reproduce the normal pulsatile pressure wave.

A convenient way to classify the pumps so far constructed is by the type of flow—whether it is basically pulsatile or nonpulsatile. The nonpulsatile pumps in common use are finger pumps and roller pumps, and most of the pulsatile pumps work by flexing a diaphragm of some sort or by using pistons.

A common type of finger pump is shown in Figure 10.3. The basic principle is to cause a tube to be closed by a series of cam-operated fingers that are arranged along the length of the tube and that successively apply pressure to the tube, thus causing the blood to move along by a sort of "milking" action. A slight amount of pulsation is produced because a small number of fingers is used (usually four or five), and the closing sequence must keep re-

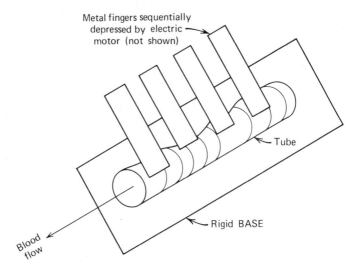

Figure 10.3   Principle of the finger pump.

cycling, causing a pressure wave instead of a continuous force. Because the fingers almost completely block the tube there is no way in which the fluid can flow backward, and therefore there is no need for valves. The fact that the blood is confined to a plastic tube simplifies sterilization procedures, because the tube may easily be sterilized separately from all other parts of the apparatus, and nothing else comes in contact with the blood.

Control of volume and pulse rate is normally accomplished by changing the speed of the motor, so that an increase in pumping volume is accompanied by an increase in pulse rate. There is a modification in which volume is controlled by the stroke length (more fingers) so that the pulse rate may be kept fixed, but in most applications a change in pulse rate does not prove to be any problem, perhaps because the pulsations are so unphysiologic in the first place.

The mechanical construction of such pumps is quite simple, although a fairly elaborate cam mechanism is necessary for the fingers. The cam mechanism is somewhat difficult to adjust for different size tubings. The weakest link in all pumps of this type, however, is the tubing itself. Experience has showed that the pressure must be applied transversely to the axis of flow: it cannot be applied longitudinally if there is to be substantial tube life. There are several methods of applying pressure to tubes, one of which is the mechanical fingers just described, but the same comments apply to other methods of squeezing tubes; these will be described subsequently. Normally, tube wear depends on the number of flexures and a heat-fatigue factor that is related to the speed of compression, the viscosity of the material to be pumped, and the presence and suitability of a lubricant. It has been stated [4] that the stress caused by the internal working of the tube material causes more damage to the tube than the wear caused by the action of the fingers. It takes about 120 lb to completely close a piece of Tygon tubing ⅛ in. thick and with an inner diameter of ½ in. A considerable amount of heat is developed by this force at 300 or 400 rpm. Fortunately, for heart pumps the fluid itself helps to dissipate the heat. Externally applied greases have been used, but they do not seem to extend tube life very much.

Hemolysis has been measured with these pumps [4]. There is some evidence that this is caused by turbulence in the blood flow and not by the pump per se. It has been suggested that if care is taken to ensure laminar flow, hemolysis will be kept at a minimum.

A natural modification of the finger pump is to use a small roller on the rim of a wheel to compress the tube, as indicated schematically in Figure 10.4. This type of pump has been used extensively in the past in blood transfusions and today is the one most commonly used for open heart surgery. It has the same advantages as the finger pump. Several rollers are usually used to reduce the rotation speed of the wheel. The blood handling portion is a tube that is easily sterilized, and the pumped volume is proportional to the motor speed. It has the advantage over the finger pumps in that it is mechanically much simpler. Its main disadvantage is that the freely rotating rollers produce shear forces, which damage the blood cells. These forces may be visualized with the help of Figure 10.2. While the roller arm is operating a friction force rotates the roller in the direction opposite to that of the roller arm, and a reaction force on the inner wall of the tubing tends to produce a movement of the tubing in the direction of rotation of the central shaft. During this "walking" of the tubing the wall in contact with the roller moves more than the outer wall. If the roller is set to completely block (or occlude) the tube, this differential movement sets up two harmful forces: a force inside the wall of the

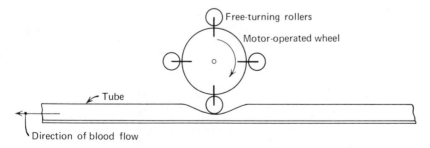

Figure 10.4 Principle of the roller pump.

tubing that causes failure at the point where the inner and outer walls meet, and an internal shear force that tends to grind the blood cells in a "mill" produced by the motion of the inner and outer walls of the blood-filled tube. There is also differential movement of the tubing walls caused directly by the force of the roller arm.

Other complications can arise because of this walking; for example, the tubing can become kinked and jammed inside the roller mechanism. Most of the undesirable results of the walking (except for the shear forces generated) can be prevented by properly attaching the tubing where it enters and leaves the pump, so that during the recycling of the roller the walls of the tube snap back to the original position.

Wesolowski [5], in an attempt to avoid the internal shear forces, has designed a roller pump that uses an internal gear arrangement, with a pinion gear locked into the roller to take up the roller's forces of rotation.

As with all pumps, hemolysis is an ever-present problem. Some of the methods that can be used with the roller pump to reduce it are as follows:

1. Use of stiff vinyl plastic tubing instead of pliable rubber tubing;
2. Increasing the diameter of the tubing in the pump head;
3. Setting the roller so it is nonocclusive;
4. Use of a lubricant at the roller-tubing interface to allow greater slippage of the roller on the tubing;
5. Use of the internal gear arrangement just described.

The use of nonocclusive settings has certain problems associated with it. If the tubing is not completely closed by the roller, the pump is no longer of the

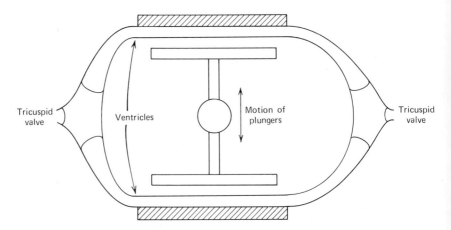

Figure 10.5 Method of operation of the Medical Monitor pump.

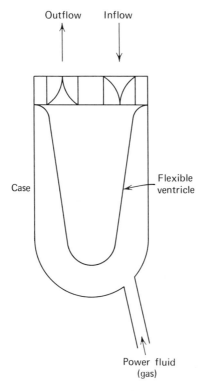

Figure 10.6   Principle behind the Army pump.

positive-displacement type, and the pump output then depends on the hydraulic resistance at the output side of the pump. If occlusive settings are used for more than a day, some provision must be made to change the tubing on the pump head, because of the danger of failure from the shear forces.

Although they have a fluctuating output pressure, the pumps just described are basically not pulsatile pumps. However, it is obviously a simple step to go from the mechanisms described for compressing the tubes to other techniques for compressing tubes that would give true pulsatile flow. In all of these pumps the tube that is being compressed is actually an artificial ventricle, and the differences between the various types of pumps are just different ways of compressing the ventricle. Two basically continuous methods have just been described, and these are mechanical. In the pulsatile pumps compression of the ventricle has been mechanical, pneumatic, and hydraulic. Examples of these three types [6] are shown schematically in the mechanical Medical Monitor pump of Figure 10.5, the pneumatic Army pump of Figure 10.6, and the hy-

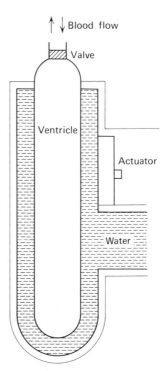

Figure 10.7   Schematic of the Davol pump.

draulic pump manufactured by Davol (Figure 10.7). The ventricles are not necessarily simple tubes now; they can be in a variety of shapes, as is clear from the illustrations. The most common and suitable materials for these tubes are polyvinylchloride and silicone rubber. Ventricles that are pneumatically and mechanically actuated depend on the elastic recoil of the walls and gravity for refilling of the chamber, which introduces the danger of fatigue of the material, and the limits of a maximum pumping rate. Valves are necessary with pumps of this type; a great variety has been used, including bicuspid, tricuspid, ball, and flap valves. Chapter 11 discusses valves in more detail.

The operation of the Davol pump, as an example of a hydraulically operated pump, is shown in Figure 10.7. This pump is a true tube pump with a straight polyvinyl tube for a ventricle with bicuspid valves at each end. The actuator is a clear Plexiglas chamber filled with water and containing the ventricle. A pneumatic piston applies force to the water, which in turn compresses the immersed ventricle, causing the blood to be propelled. The blood flows in the proper direction because of the valves. The stroke ercursion of the piston is set manually and is variable from 0 to 60 ml. This type of pump has been used principally in open heart operations. The rate is variable from 30 to 200 per minute, but it may be synchronized in certain applications with the R wave from the electrocardiogram, since a discrete action (motion of the piston) initiates each heartbeat. It has been used for "counterpulsation," in which the assist device beats synchronously with the natural heart. It takes much of the load by aspirating blood during systole and returning it to the arterial tree during diastole [14]. Synchronization is accomplished by sensing the R wave and using it to trigger the pump. It responds automatically to changes in flow by means of an ingenious fluid-amplifier system and has a relatively nontraumatic pulsatile flow because of its pneumatic compression.

The fluid-amplifier system in the device reproduces the function of the human heart with reasonable accuracy, but the whole device has no electronics and only eight moving parts—four heart valves, two ventricles, and two suction-control flappers. The heart has two pumping chambers fastened together. Each pump consists of a plastic shell that houses a ventricle and a metal header that holds the ventricle in its housing also positions the bicuspid valves above the ventricles.

The Medical Monitor pump is a tube pump that is activated by shoes on an eccentric cam, somewhat similar in idea to the roller pump. Stroke volume and flow depend on the output hydraulic resistance, and variation of output flow is adjusted by changing the rate, as in the roller pumps. The stroke volume is small, as is also true of the roller pump.

The pumps that have been described up to now have usually been used during open heart operations for short-term assistance. Most of the pumps that have been proposed for implantation are diaphragm pumps, and in general these have been pneumatically operated. It is necessary to be somewhat careful in definitions here, because if the term "diaphragm pump" were used to include any pump with one or more flexible walls, then almost all of the types of pumps discussed so far could be included. For the purposes of this discussion a diaphragm pump is a flexible-walled container that is activated by liquid or gas that is constrained on one surface by an inflexible chamber.

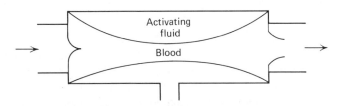

Figure 10.8   One of the four types of heart pumps.

Diaphragm pumps are operated principally by liquid or gas. Liquid has the advantage of being noncompressible, which allows more accurate control of diaphragm motion. This, however, is not a great advantage and is offset by the necessity for pumping liquid through tubes and of having to maintain a supply of the liquid. Air, on the other hand, is always available and is as efficient as liquid if the conduit is only a few feet, as is the case with all present pumps whose source of motive power is external to the body.

The situation might change considerably if a totally implanted power source for an artificial heart were developed. Air would not be available, because to obtain some the body would have to be opened at some point for a tube to pass through. Thus the driving

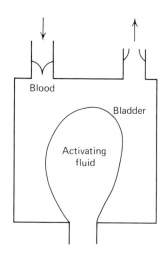

Figure 10.9 Another type of heart pump.

medium would have to be enclosed in an internal reservoir, from where it would be transmitted only a short distance to the actual pump mechanism. In this case the greater density and efficiency of a liquid medium would permit smaller size and less power consumption. Some diaphragm pumps have been designed to work directly from electricity without any intervening medium, but these are not so well developed as the pneumatic and hydraulic ones.

Most diaphragm-pump artificial hearts fall into one of four categories:

1. A flexible, blood-filled tube is contained in a rigid container, as illustrated in Figure 10.8. Liquid or gas is forced into the space between the tube and the container, causing the tube-shaped ventricle to fill and empty, and valves at the end control the direction of flow.

2. A flexible bladder extends into a rigid, blood-filled container, as illustrated in Figure 10.9. Liquid or gas is forced into the bladder. This was essentially the design of one of the earliest practical heart pumps, that of Dale and Schuster, first described in 1928.

3. The converse of (2); that is, a blood-filled flexible bladder encased in a rigid container, as illustrated in Figure 10.10. The flow is similar to that of the tubular pump of (1). This is essentially the design of the Kolff and DeBakey pumps, as well as a number of others. In most of these designs the outer container has been of deformable plastic, but this plastic has been relatively inelastic; that is, it can be easily bent, but not easily stretched.

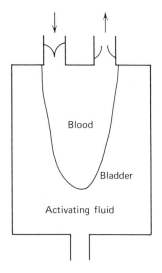

Figure 10.10 Third type of heart pump.

4. A conventional pump of the diaphragm type (Figure 10.11) has blood on one side of the diaphragm and liquid or gas on the other.

These figures are all intended to be schematic, not representative of any one particular design. Note that the difference between a tube-compression pump and a diaphragm–pump is often more a matter of definition than a difference in operating principles.

Probably the most important advantage of existing diaphragm pumps is that they propel suitable volumes of blood at physiological pressures and rates with very little damage to the blood, perhaps because the action of a diaphragm pump is similar to that of the natural heart. We would expect, on this basis, that a pump with only flexible walls in contact with the blood would produce less damage to red blood cells than a pump with rigid walls.

All of these pumps inherently produce a pulsatile flow whose waveform can be controlled to be almost identical to that of the heart. The waveform is adjusted by controlling the activating fluid or gas.

The fact that the characteristics of the pump can be regulated quite closely

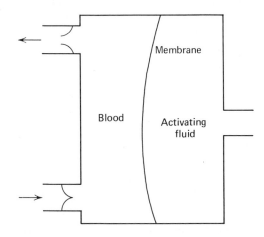

Figure 10.11   A fourth type of membrane heart pump.

by controlling the pumping fluid (liquid or gas) provides some valuable fringe benefits. Thus it is possible to have the stroke volume regulated by the venous return, which is an advantage because venous return can almost disappear under certain circumstances, whereas it can increase greatly during exercise. Also, the fact that the intraventricular pressure during diastole can be regulated can be used to hold venous pressure as well as arterial pressure at physiologic levels.

The size of the pump can be made to approximate that of the heart itself very closely, and the stroke volume can be made the same as that of a natural heart in about the same volume. The shape is also extremely flexible.

Note, however, that with a heart of this type, at the present state of the art, the pumping mechanism may be the smallest part of the whole device. A pump that operates on compressed air needs an air compressor, and at the present time these are quite large. Similarly, a hydraulic pump requires a fluid reservoir and a secondary pump to move the fluid.

In addition to hemolysis, some of the disadvantages of the diaphragm pumps are that they require valves, which increases the blood cell damage, and that they contain more moving parts, which can break. Also, fairly stiff tubes must pass through the chest wall to connect the heart with the external driving mechanism. A motor-driven pump or the electrically operated piezoelectric pump, which will be described later, require only thin, flexible wires. A totally implanted power source would, of course, eliminate this problem.

From a reliability standpoint leaks are probably a much bigger problem with this type of pump than with the others. If a leak is present with a hydraulic pump, the fluid will eventually all be lost, and the pump will be unable to operate. Although this is not true with a pneumatic pump, leaks cut down on the pressure head. This would not be too serious with a large air compressor, but it would be a major problem with an implanted source that could generate just enough power to operate the device. Leaks would be especially dangerous if they occurred in the diaphragm itself, because this would cause contamination of the blood by the hydraulic fluid and eventual catastrophic rupture of the diaphragm. Unfortunately, the diaphragm is most vulnerable to leakage because it is subject to the greatest stress.

Artificial hearts that have been designed by various investigators will now be described briefly, not to give a detailed discussion of all of the factors that may make one design superior to another (although some of these may be indicated), but to give enough detail for the reader to appreciate the present state of the art.

An artificial heart that has served as a model for others is the one developed by Kolff at the Cleveland Clinic [7–9] (see Figure 10.12). It is basically two pumps, one for each side of the heart, of the type with a rigid outer case

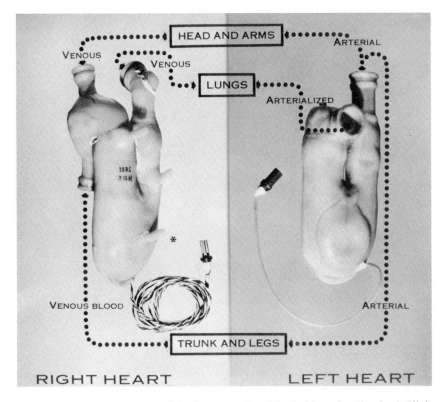

Figure 10.12 Operation of artificial heart developed by Kolff at the Cleveland Clinic Foundation. (Courtesy of the National Institutes of Health.)

and a flexible Silastic sac inside, and it looks something like a natural heart. The motive force is supplied by compressed air. This heart has been implanted in a calf, that survived for 2 days. As with many other devices of this type, the air compressor and control equipment is not implanted but is external to the body.

The materials used are medical-grade silicone rubber for the ventricles, Lexan for the ventricle housings, anodized aluminum for the valve headers, and polyethylene for the valves. The basic principles of this type of control were tested on the Army artificial heart pump. Although the Army pump is an external device, the same type of control problems exist. Tests on this pump demonstrated that it was able to maintain arterial pressures when there was adequate venous return and to respond properly to changes in venous pressure.

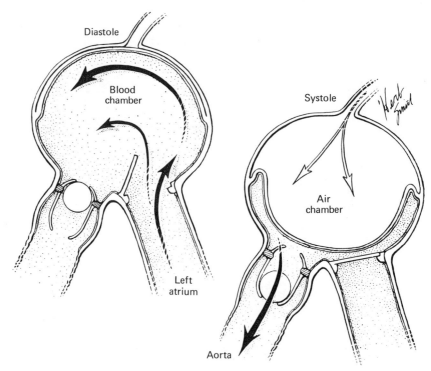

Figure 10.13   Membrane heart pump. (Courtesy of the National Institutes of Health.)

Another implantable heart that is quite widely known and has been used in humans is that of DeBakey and his associates [10]. It is actually an implantable pump used to bypass the left ventricle and is used only as a temporary method of providing rest for the heart. Here, too, the entire power mechanism is too large to be placed inside the body. It is also of the pneumatic diaphragm type (see Figure 10.13), fabricated from Dacron-reinforced silicone rubber with ball valves at the inlet and outlet to ensure unidirectional flow. It is coupled to the external power and controlling system by means of ¼-in. outside diameter tubes. Compressed carbon dioxide is pulsed into the gas chamber, causing the central blood chamber to collapse and empty. The inlet of the pump is connected to the left atrium, and the outlet is connected to the descending aorta through a woven Dacron tube graft. More examples are shown in Figure 10.14. As may be seen, blood passing through the pump bypasses the left ventricle.

The external power and control system consists of a Teflon bellows driven by an electric motor. A control system initiates the pump cycle in response to

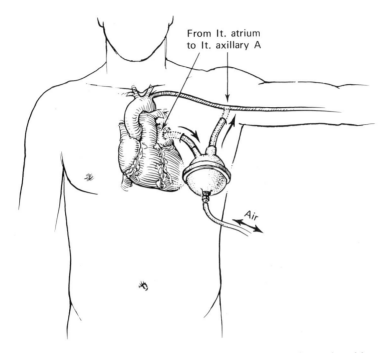

Figure 10.14 Left ventricular bypass designed at Baylor and Rice Universities capable of taking over most of the workload of a damaged or failing human heart for a limited period of time. (Courtesy of the National Institutes of Health.)

an electrocardiographic signal. Motor speed control is provided by silicon controlled rectifiers, and a dynamic braking circuit stops the motor completely at the end of each stroke. The system can maintain synchronization either with every electrocardiogram (ECG) cycle, every other cycle, or every third one. This part of the device also ensures continuous (although possibly unsynchronized) operation if the ECG rate becomes very high or is interrupted. Another means of synchronizing the pump is to use a pressure signal from the left atrium instead of an ECG signal. A recent modification of this device is the use of a plastic "velour" lining in the ventricles, which minimizes blood-cell damage and clot formation by rapid formation of a pseudointima.

A similar idea, but with different mechanization, has been tested in humans by Kantrowitz [11, 12]. Again the purpose is to supply a temporary-assist pump, but in series with the left ventricle, instead of in parallel with it. This device is also a pneumatic diaphragm–pump; the ventricle consists of a flexible inner dynamic bulb in a partly rigid outer shell of the same shape, both made of Dacron-reinforced silicone rubber (Figure 10.15). A large

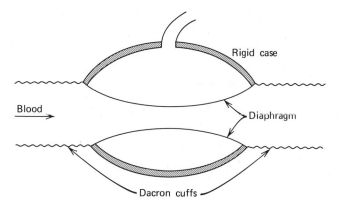

Figure 10.15   Auxiliary ventricle developed by Kantrowitz.

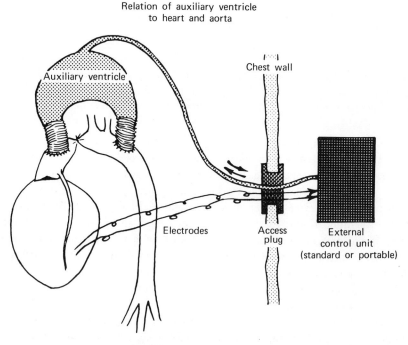

Figure 10.16   Method of using Kantrowitz's auxiliary ventricle in actual implantation. (Courtesy of the National Institutes of Health.)

woven Dacron tube about 0.5 in. in diameter is bonded to each end of inner bulb. The system has no valves; proper unidirectional flow is maintained by synchronizing the action of the pump with that of the left ventricle, as determined by the ECG signals. The pumping bulb has a volume of about 15 ml, which is half the stroke volume of the ventricle of a 35-lb dog.

The device is implanted by fastening one Dacron cuff to the ascending aorta and the other cuff to the descending aorta. The ascending aorta is then blocked between the connections, so that the entire output of the ventricle passes through the pumping chamber (Figure 10.16). The ventricle is driven by compressed air, brought from the exterior through a tube to the space between the inner and outer bulbs. The air flow is interrupted by an electronically controlled valve, which is in turn regulated ultimately by the R wave of the left ventricle. The air tube and electrodes pass through the skin to the outside power source and timing circuit. The timing is adjusted so that the pump fills at the beginning of systole of the left ventricle, thus lowering the latter's outflow resistance and reducing its work at the end of systole; the aortic valve closes naturally, and air is forced into the artificial ventricle, expelling the blood. Thus the heart's own valves are used to ensure that the blood goes in the right direction. This is possible only because the artificial ventricle is in series with the natural one, instead of being in parallel, as is the case with most of the other artificial hearts.

Clinical studies in dogs indicate a 40- to 60-percent reduction in left ventricle work. It is intended that the auxiliary ventricle remain permanently implanted in the body and that the patient be connected to the power source either in case of a heart attack or on some scheduled basis. It still remains to be demonstrated if aiding only the left side of the heart will produce enough improvement to be worthwhile—or if it is in fact necessary to boost both sides of the heart, as is done by Kolff's device.

The principal problem with all of these pumps is that a large external source of power is required, and tubing of some sort is needed to bring the activating medium into the body. Motor driven piston-type pumps do not have this problem, but in general the piston action has turned out to be damaging to blood cells. For this reason a diaphragm pump that operates directly from electricity is of considerable interest, even if it is not now practical. The best known example of this type of pump is one developed by Loehr and his associates [13, 14], based on the piezoelectric effect. In asymmetric crystals such as Rochelle salt and barium titanate, and also in certain ceramics, an applied electric field produces mechanical motion, and, conversely, applied motion produces an electric field. Such devices are the basis for crystal phonograph pickups and crystal microphones, and are also the power-generating portion of a biologically powered pacemaker described elsewhere in this book.

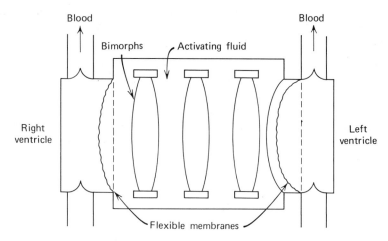

Figure 10.17　Basic principal of piezoelectric pump. (After Loehr.)

The direction of the displacement depends on the electric field direction, and the amplitude depends on the field intensity. These materials are efficient converters of electrical to mechanical energy, and vice versa.

An oil pump that depends on this principle has been used since 1958. The pump has no moving parts, but instead uses concentric cylinders of a piezoelectric ceramic. It was discovered that this particular pump could not be used to handle blood, because the applied frequency (which is the frequency at which the piezoelectric plates vibrate) was so high that the blood cells were damaged. The Loehr device works at the low cardiac frequencies, using "bimorphs" to increase the motion of the piezoelectric materials. A bimorph consists of two sheets of piezoelectric ceramic cemented together and oriented so that as one expands the other contracts, causing the sheet to bend. The movement of the bulging surface depends on the material and the dimensions of the disk. Figure 10.17 shows how these disks may be used to make a pump. The disks themselves are mounted in rubber suspension rings that minimize peripheral restraint. Alternate cells are connected together, and an intermediate fluid is pumped against flexible ventricles of the tube type previously discussed, which are at the ends of the column. Thus this device is really two diaphragm pumps in series: one uses piezoelectric plates and pumps the intermediate fluid; the other used silicone rubber and pumps the blood. The construction used results in one integrated device that still has no moving parts and requires only an electrical input. Since the pressure waveform depends on the electrical waveform, it is quite easy to control.

Even if this heart is used, it would still be necessary to get electrical energy into the body by some means. Wires, or any other material passing through an opening in the skin, are focal points for infection and are in general unsatisfactory for long-term applications. Methods for providing power to implanted devices are discussed in a later chapter.

REFERENCES

[1] Salisbury, P., "Physiology of Assisted Circulation," *Mechanical Devices to Assist the Failing Heart,* NAS Publication No. 1283, 1966, p. 3.

[2] Opinions expressed on pulsatile flow are those of the authors. Much of the technical data may be found in the following: Varco, R., E. Bernstein, A. Costanoda, and P. Blackshear, "Physiologic Problems in Prolonged Pumping," *Mechanical Devices to Assist the Failing Heart,* op. cit., p. 45.

[3] Rainer, W. G., "Pulsatile versus Nonpulsatile Pumping," ibid., p. 59.

[4] Hungerford, V. G., "Finger Pumps," ibid., p. 73.

[5] Wesolowski, S., "Roller Pumps," ibid., p. 77.

[6] Lefenine, A., and D. Harken, "Tube Compression Pumps," ibid., p. 86.

[7] Nosé, L., S. Topaz, A. Sengupth, C. Tretbar, and W. Kolff, "Artificial Hearts Inside the Pericardial Sac in Calves," *Trans. ASAIO,* 11:255 (1965).

[8] Woodward, K., H. Straub, Y. Nosé, and W. Kolff, "An Intrathoracic Artificial Heart Controlled by Fluid Amplifiers," *Trans. ASAIO,* 12:294 (1966).

[9] Nosé, Y., C. Sarin, M. Klain, K. Leitz, T. Teony, P. Phillips, F. Rose, and W. Kolff, "Elimination of Some Problems Encountered in Total Replacement of the Heart with an Intrathoracic Mechanical Pump: Venous Return," *Trans. ASAIO,* 12:301 (1966).

[10] DeBakey, M., D. Liotta, and C. W. Hall, "Left-Heart Bypass Using an Implantable Blood Pump," *Mechanical Devices to Assist the Failing Heart,* op. cit., p. 223.

[11] Kantrowiz, A. (in discussion), ibid., p. 208.

[12] U.S. Department of Health, Education, and Welfare, *Fact Sheet Artificial Parts for the Heart and Blood Vessels,* 1967.

[13] Loehr, M., W. Kosch, M. Suges, and G. Danielson (in discussion), ibid., p. 133.

[14] Loehr, M., W. Kosch, M. Singer, W. Pierce, and C. Kirby, "The Piezoelectric Artificial Heart," *Trans. ASAIO,* 10:147 (1964).

CHAPTER ELEVEN

Passive Implants

The general categories of implanted devices in the body were discussed in the first chapter, where it was pointed out that these devices could be roughly divided into active and passive implants. The active implant has some form of energy input (and therefore usually an energy output in some form), and the passive implant is basically structural in nature (e.g., a conduit of some type or an internal splint).

1. CATEGORIES OF PASSIVE IMPLANTS

It is convenient to consider the passive implants according to the parts of the body in which they are used, because structurally and chemically many of them are similar. They can be divided into seven broad classes: cardiovascular, respiratory, digestive, genitourinary, nervous, miscellaneous senses, and miscellaneous soft tissues. Only the devices that are in use or seem to be feasible in the near future are considered. This chapter is an outline of these devices, rather than a detailed discussion.

Cardiovascular System

The most important passive cardiovascular prosthetics are heart valves, heart walls, and arteries. The heart valve is somewhat on the borderline between active and passive, because it actually has an energy input from the blood flow and an output that is the modulated flow of blood through the heart. Heart-wall prostheses are basically "patches," and artificial arteries are tubes. Artificial arteries may be made from plastic or from transplanted tissue, either from the same person or from another person (or animal). Although transplanted tissues are important and are widely used, they are outside the scope of this book, which considers only synthetic organs.

Respiratory System

The important replacements to be considered here are the artificial larynx, trachea, bronchus, and chest wall. These are examples both of structural replacements and conduits.

Digestive System

Both an artificial esophagus and an artificial bile duct have been used. Both are conduits.

Genitourinary System

Although the external artificial kidney is a well-developed device, implanted artificial kidneys are yet to come. Passive implants in the genitourinary system have been mainly the ureter and the urethra, again conduits.

Nervous System

An actual operating artificial neuron is not yet in sight (although the synchronous pacemaker might be considered a primitive form of one). Nervous system prostheses are mainly supports and conduits, and include artificial dura (the membrane covering the spinal cord and brain), tubing to shunt fluids in hydrocephalus, and sprayed plastics used as supports for aneurysms (dilatations of arteries).

Sensory Systems

Various synthetic devices have been used for the eye and ear, such as the artificial lens and cornea. The artificial glass eye is probably one of the oldest of prosthetic devices, but unfortunately it is mainly cosmetic, not functional.

Miscellaneous Soft Tissues

Plastic meshes have been used with considerable success in repairing hernias. Artificial tendons have been used with some success also. Silicone fluids have been used to separate parts that might adhere and grow together. Here the synthetic is used as a lubricant and may be considered more of a drug than a prosthetic.

The basic principles in the design of these devices have been already covered, but it is useful to review each of these devices in detail.

2. ARTIFICIAL VALVES

A typical present day heart valve is basically a silicone rubber ball in a metal cage, as shown in Figure 11.1. Positive pressure on the inflow port pushes the ball against the cage, allowing the blood to pass through. Negative pressure sucks the ball against the port, preventing backflow. The first successful implanted artificial valve was developed by Hufnagel: it was placed in the descending thoracic aorta. This device was a ball valve in a Lucite

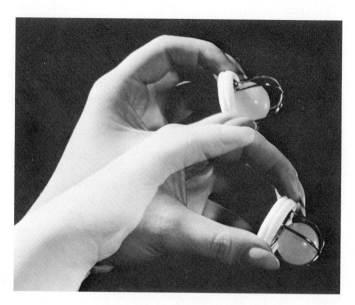

Figure 11.1   The Starr-Edwards ball valve which has been used to replace natural mitral valves. (Courtesy of the National Institutes of Health.)

housing. The aortic ends fitted tightly around the housing and were held in place by serrated rings.

This valve, although similar in construction to present day valves, had many disadvantages in addition to these still existing in all heart valves. It was noisy, so much so that some patients threatened to commit suicide rather than hear the persistent "beating" of the valves; and because heart lung machines were not yet in use, the valve could only be placed in the thoracic aorta, too far downstream to really do the job intended.

Significant improvements in the aortic valve were made by Starr, and the extensive experience with this valve (known as the Starr-Edwards valve) has resulted in significant success. Starr's value has a metal ball-retaining cage made of highly polished molded cobalt-chromium-molybdenum alloy, known as Stellite 21, that is hard and resistant to corrosion and mechanical wear, and does not predispose to clotting of the blood. A solid ball of silicone rubber is held within the cage, and a cuff of knitted Teflon is attached to the metal ring so that it may be sutured to the aortic ring.

There are still some problems with this valve. In 10 to 15 percent of cases clots develop at the junction between the textile and the metal. Davila [1] attempted to overcome this by making the metallic surface rough, so that it becomes coated with fibrin and presumably becomes coated with endothelium, and more recently the struts have also been covered with Teflon cloth. The valve seat also becomes covered with tissue, so that the seat can maintain its shape only because of the repeated impact of the ball. Clinical experience with this type of valve is still being gathered.

A significant pressure drop can occur across the valve when it is opened during systole because the valve seat and attachment ring make the opening smaller than the natural aortic ring. If the cage is too large to compensate for this, it will protrude into the aorta, so that when the ball enters the cage it obstructs flow.

Cartwright [2] attempted to solve the problem by using a double-cage valve in which the ball seats inside the opening and thus the travel into the aorta is less, although the total excursion is about the same. In this device the plunger is lenticular instead of spherical, which shortens the valve still more. This principle has been incorporated into a number of other valves.

Another valve, designed by Magovern [3], is fixed in place by metallic pins that bite into the valve ring at the time of implantation and hold the valve in place. This method permits the valve to be implanted quickly and reduces the time required on the heart-lung pump.

Ball valves have also been used successfully for mitral valve replacement,

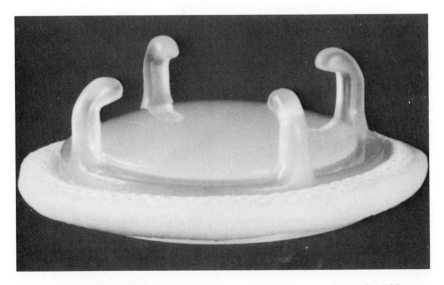

Figure 11.2 Hufnagel Discoid valve, an example of a floating disk valve. (Courtesy of the National Institutes of Health.)

but there is a higher incidence of clot formation than for the aortic value. In this location the pressure drop across the valve is small because the valve port is quite large.

Many other types of valves are being tested, including flaps, plungers, and discs (Figures 11.2, 11.3, and 11.4), all designed with the intent of diminishing clot formation and enlarging the valve orifice. There is as yet insufficient clinical evidence to indicate the clear superiority of any of these.

Although various complications, including clot formation and red cell damage, occur with all types of valves, there is no doubt that artificial valves can replace the natural valves for long periods of time.

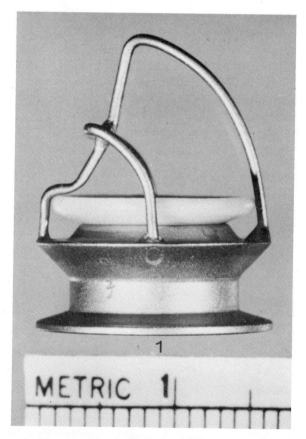

Figure 11.3   Cruz-Kaster valve features a meniscus-shaped disk. During forward flow the disk tips upward, thus providing a maximum orifice and offering minimum resistance to flow. (Courtesy of the National Institutes of Health.)

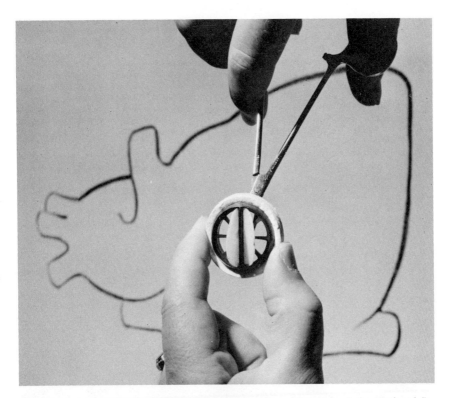

Figure 11.4 Gott-Daggett hinged leaflet mitral valve. (Courtesy of the National Institutes of Health.)

Another approach to valve design is to imitate the natural valve by using flexible leaflets. Efforts to date have not been successful. If porous material is used (such as textiles), the leaflets become thick and stiff after the fabric becomes infiltrated with fibrous tissue. Nonporous leaflets, on the other hand, tend to form clots. (Recently, grafted tissue leaflets from cadavers have had some success.)

3. HEART-WALL REPAIR AND ARTIFICIAL ARTERIES

Artificial materials have been used to repair defects in the outer wall of the heart and in the septa between the chambers [4, 5, 6]. Compressed Ivalon was one of the earliest materials used, but it tended to become rigid and brittle with time. Fabrics, which do not have this problem, are prefer-

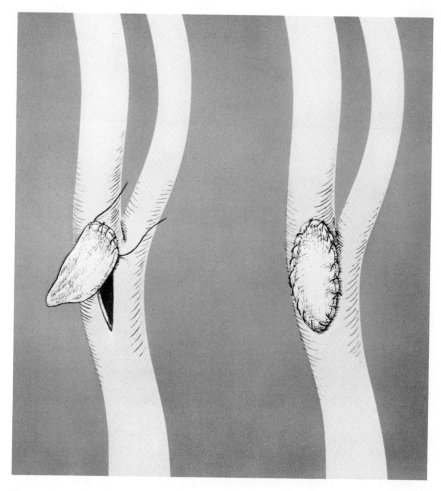

Figure 11.5   Use of artificial patch material to reconstruct a blood vessel after it has been opened for removal of fatty deposits. (Courtesy of the National Institutes of Health.)

able, especially when knitted. Teflon and Dacron are excellent materials because they are strong, nonreactive, noncarcinogenic, and tend to retain tensile strength indefinitely. Such patches are rarely more than 2 cm in diameter, and as a result healing complications are rare. These patches are illustrated in Figure 11.5.

Similarly, arterial prostheses are made from Dacron and Teflon cloth as shown in Figure 11.6. These materials become completely incorporated into

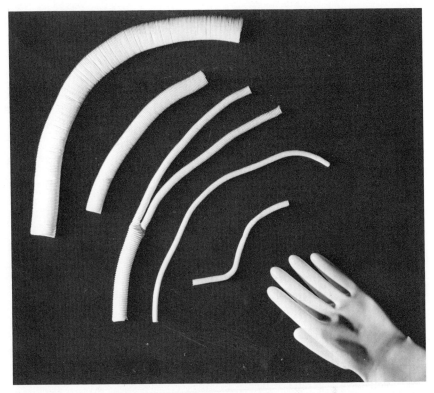

Figure 11.6 Various types and sizes of vascular prostheses. (Courtesy of the National Institutes of Health.)

the body by virtue of invasion of the interstices of the cloth with fibrous tissue and formation of a pseudointima. Experience has shown that such artificial arteries are highly reliable and in general will outlive the patient. Arteries have been transplanted from one human to another, but these grafts tend to fail early and therefore are no longer used. Further discussion of such homografts (man to man) and heterografts (animal to man) is beyond the scope of this text.

At first, solid-walled tubes of glass and various metals were used to repair arteries, but obstruction of the flow by clot formation and rupture of the graft at the junction with the host vessel occurred often. The feasibility of porous plastic tubes was first demonstrated by Voorhees. The more porous a material is, the more readily it is accepted by the body; the upper limit to porosity, measured with water, is approximately 5000 ml/min-cm^2 at a pressure of 120 mm Hg. This is the upper limit with respect to bleeding at time of implantation [4]. However, it has been shown that if it were not for the problem of bleeding at time of implantation, a porosity of up to 10,000 ml/min-cm^2 would result in superior acceptance of the prosthesis. One way of solving this problem is to have a material which has a different porosity at time of implant (the "implant porosity") and after it is in place (the "biological" porosity). One way of doing this is to have a material in the interstices of the mesh which is adsorbed by the body, thus producing a low porosity at implantation but a high porosity after implantation. One such fabrication uses Dacron as a matrix and collagen as a resorbable component. Its porosity at implant can be as low as 20 ml/min-cm^2 at implant, but it has gone up to 5000 ml/min-cm^2 during healing [7].

Characteristics that are desirable in vascular prostheses are the following:

1. No toxicity, allergenicity, or other chemical reactions.

2. Durability without deterioration after long implantation.

3. Porosity, measured with water, of 5000 ml/min-cm^2 and an implant porosity of less than 50 ml/min-cm^2.

4. Linear elasticity. Crimping is a desirable configuration because it permits flexion of the material without buckling and obstruction of flow.

5. Pliability and twistability.

There are very few prostheses that meet all of these characteristics. The porosity requirements are difficult to meet. If the graft is too porous, blood will be lost through the graft walls. If the material is not porous enough, the graft will have a greater tendency to produce clots.

Wesolowski and his co-workers [4] have attempted to develop a "compound" prosthesis using both absorbable and permanent materials. They tested open-mesh fabrics coated with collagen (a body protein); woven fabrics in which some of the polyester yarns are replaced with monofilament yarns of catgut; and fabrics woven of a yarn with a compound core, where the core is monofilament collofil (a type of catgut) and a multifilament of polyester yarn is wrapped around the core. These grafts diminished the porosity at implantation by a factor of 100, but in other respects they behaved much as standard cloth prostheses. These artificial grafts are still undergoing testing.

Parsonnet has approached this problem by preforming collagen tubes in the recipient animal. Silicone rods wrapped in Dacron mesh were inserted under the skin of dogs 5 or more weeks before use. On removing the rod it was found that collagen had impregnated the mesh to form a natural protein tube supported by the mesh. These tubes have been used successfully in animals but have not been tested in humans.

Venous grafts are not nearly as successful as arterial grafts. Clots form readily in all vein grafts because the blood flow in veins is slow. Attempts have been made to prevent this by applying a negative charge to the vein walls or by using nonthrombogenic plastics, such as graphite-benzylkonium-heparin and similar materials discussed in the section on plastics. The ultimate graft will probably be developed from this type of material.

REFERENCES

[1] Davila, J., "Development of Artificial Heart Valves," *Plastics in Surgery Implants*, ASTM Special Publication No. 383, 1965, p. 1.

[2] Cartwright, R., E. Smeloff, T. Davey, and B. Kaufman, "Development of a Titanium Double-Caged Full Orifice Ball Valve," *Trans. ASAIO*, 10:231 (1964).

[3] Magovern, G., and H. Cromie, "Sutureless Prosthetic Heart Valve," *J. Thor. and Cardiovas. Surg.*, 46:726 (1963).

[4] Wesolowski, S., A. Martinez, and O. McMahon, "Use of Artificial Materials in Surgery," *Current Problems in Surgery*, Yearbook Medical Publishers, Chicago, December, 1966.

[5] U. S. Department of Health, Education, and Welfare, *Fact Sheet Artificial Parts for the Heart and Blood Vessels*, 1967.

[6] American Society for Testing Materials, *Plastics in Surgical Implants*, ASTM Special Publication No. 386, 1965.

[7] Liebig, W. "Fundamental Problems in Development of Prosthetic Vascular Grafts," in *Fundamentals of Vascular Grafting*, S. Wesolowski and C. Dennis, Eds., p. 129. Blakiston Div. of McGraw-Hill, New York, 1963.

CHAPTER TWELVE

Other Energy Sources

The previous discussions of implanted devices that require power to operate them, including the pacemaker and the artificial heart, have indicated the great importance of their sources of power. The lack of suitable implanted power sources prevents the pacemaker from running indefinitely, and presently there is no power source that could be implanted for an artificial heart. Thus it is not surprising that the field of power sources for implantable prosthetics is an active field of research. At present, only two sources of power are used to any considerable degree for pacemakers: either implantable batteries or power transmitted through the skin by means of radio energy. Experimental artificial hearts use either direct wires (or air lines) through the skin or some form of electromagnetic induction. Attempts to remove the dependence of the implanted devices on these sources of power, in their present forms, are discussed in this chapter.

1. PACEMAKERS

All pacemakers currently in clinical use derive their energy from chemical cells. This is true even of the pacemakers that transmit power by radio energy, because the external device in these cases also gets its power from chemical batteries. These batteries are basically of conventional design, although they are manufactured under exacting quality-control procedures. The present life of a pacemaker with an implanted battery is on the order of 2 years, although some fail earlier, and some last much longer.

Special pacemakers with extra circuitry, such as the synchronous and standby units, tend to have somewhat shorter life. The battery life of the radio-powered pacemakers tends to be shorter still, about 1 year, because much of the energy is wasted in transmission through the skin; however, this is not so important because the batteries may be easily replaced. Induction coupled pacers (with no carrier) have shorter lives. It would seem that the radio-powered pacemaker is the ideal solution to the problem of pacemaker life, because with these devices battery replacement is simple. From a strictly technical viewpoint this is true, but it turns out that many (if not most) patients prefer an implanted pacemaker, even though they know it will have to be replaced every few years, because they do not like to wear, hanging from a belt, a device on which their life depends. Although the external device is waterproof, it seems to present a psychological barrier to many activities, especially in the case of those who engage in rather vigorous pursuits. However, it seems to offer definite advantages for children. For the above reason much effort is being expended on new power sources, especially chemical, mechanical, and thermodynamic ones.

Mechanical sources of energy generally make use of the natural movements of some parts of the body to produce electricity by means of a generator of some sort. One obvious approach is to put a turbine generator of some sort in the blood stream. The previous discussion of damage to blood cells caused by artificial hearts and valves suggests that clotting and hemolysis of blood would be the main restrictions, because damage to the blood cells would probably be great. Other problems associated with this device, such as locating the turbine where the blood velocity would be great enough and yet the circulation would not be unduly impeded, have prevented this approach from being followed.

The mechanical approach, making use of the piezoelectric effect, has proved able to operate a pacemaker. This effect has already been discussed as applied to the piezoelectric plates, which flexed to propel blood. The same effect may be used in the reverse manner to generate electricity: if the plates are flexed, they will produce electricity. The amount produced is not large, but the saving grace of all of the methods described here is that the pacemaker requires only 10 to 20 mW.

Two approaches have generated sufficient power to power a pacemaker. One of these, developed by the authors [1, 2], is illustrated in Figure 12.1. The basic transducer consists of two plates of piezoelectric ceramic (PZT–5) $1\frac{1}{4}$ by $\frac{1}{2}$ in., mounted in a cantilever fashion. The source of power is the expansion and contraction of the aorta, which lies between the free ends of the cantilevered plates. These plates (or bimorphs) generate electricity when they are bent. The open-circuit voltage produced from a dog's aorta is 10 to 20 volts. Since the capacitance of each plate is about 0.03 microfarads, the entire device stores about 6 microjoules with each heartbeat.

Four plates (two complete transducer units) were necessary to operate the pacemaker circuit of Figure 12.2, which is a modification of the General Electric pacemaker circuit. It consists basically of an *npn-pnp* transistor multivibrator with a matching transformer. A basic problem with this device is the high impedance of the transducer and the low impedance of the heart. To be efficient there must be good impedance matching; this is impractical

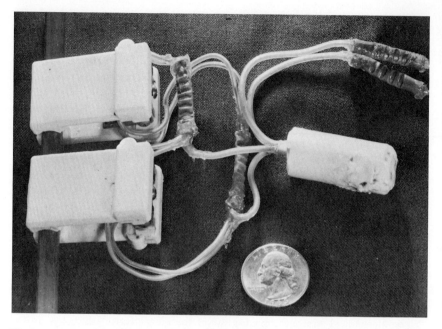

Figure 12.1 A piezoelectric generator developed by authors with accompanying encapsulated circuitry. Two generators are shown, with a tube passing where the aorta would ordinarily be.

at the 1-Hz frequency at which the heart is generating the power, but it does become practical at pulse frequencies. Therefore the entire circuit is built to operate with high-impedance components. (The resistors all have values between 10 and 15 MΩ.)

The output waveform of this circuit is a portion of an exponential, not a square pulse. The capacitors used in the rectifier circuit can store enough electricity for about 10 pulses, so that the device will continue to work even if one of the pulses is ineffective. (Indeed, the circuit cannot be made to work without this feature. If the size of the capacitors is reduced to lower the amount of charge stored—which tends to increase the output voltage—the circuit will operate as an amplifier, not a pacemaker. It produces an output pulse immediately after each heartbeat places a charge on the filter condensers.) The energy storage in the filter capacitors provides the necessary delay between the heartbeat, which generates the electricity, and the electrical pulse, which causes the heart to beat. Thus extra storage is available for pacemaker impulses.

Another device that has made use of the piezoelectric effect is illustrated

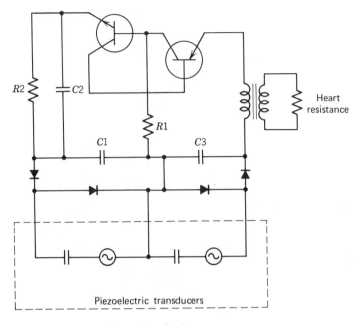

Pacemaker circuit

Figure 12.2   Details of electronic circuit used with the device in Figure 12.1.

in Figure 12.3 [3]. In this device the piezoelectric crystals are mounted behind a diaphragm in the capsule, and the capsule itself is mounted so that
the heart strikes it when it beats, thus hitting the crystal and producing electricity. The capsule must be carefully placed. If the force is too great, the
crystals will break; whereas if it is too small, insufficient electricity will be
generated. It is also questionable whether the heart will continue to strike
the crystals over a long period of time, because adaptation may cause the heart
to change its mode of expansion and contraction so that it does not hit the
crystals.

The chief problem with both of these devices has not been the general
conception, or the amount of energy, but the basic difficulty of encapsulation.
Even a small amount of moisture entering the case will materially reduce
the output of the crystals. All plastics are permeable to water vapor and are
therefore unsuitable for the flexible encapsulation needed. Metal encapsulation would appear to be the answer, but, because the crystals must bend, it
is difficult to accomplish. A solution to this problem now appears in sight.
The design of the first device shown (Figure 12.1) has been modified so
that the crystals are completely enclosed in welded metal cans and the mo-

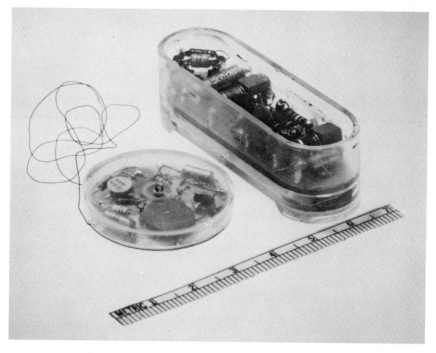

Figure 12.3   Another form of piezoelectric-powered pacemaker developed at West-ern Reserve University. The motion of the heart strikes crystals in this device. (Cour-tesy of the National Institutes of Health.)

tion of the aorta is transmitted to them through a metal bellows, which is also welded to the can. Thus a watertight seal is obtained, and a bending motion can be transmitted. The bellows reduces the power output by 10 to 20 percent, but the implanted generator has an indefinite life. If care is taken to wrap the aorta with Dacron cloth, there seems to be no problem with damage to it, and power continues to be produced. Long-term use of this device in animals is in progress. This modification is shown in Figure 12.4.

Pacemakers have also been devised to use the body as a battery [4, 5, 6]. The body fluids are electrolytes, so all that is necessary to generate electricity is to place two dissimilar metals in contact with the body tissues, and elec-tricity will be generated. There have been several demonstrations that more than enough power is available to power a pacemaker, and indeed the major considerations in this area are not technological. Many batteries produce electricity by corroding their electrodes. If such a device were used in the body, the corrosion products, some of which are toxic, would be in the body.

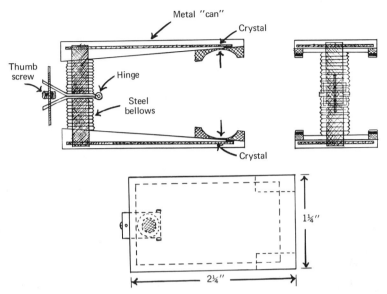

Figure 12.4 Method of encapsulating generators of the type shown in Figure 12.1 entirely in metal to permit watertight seals. Bellows transmits motion to crystal.

An attempt to circumvent this was to make the electrodes out of platinum and platinum black, neither of which corrodes. Unfortunately, the difference in the electrochemical positions of these electrodes is small, so that there is barely enough power to operate a pacemaker. If metals farther apart are used, either corrosion products or gases are released into the body. Thus application of this principle must await determination of the long-term biological effects of these by-products. Clearly, it is not satisfactory to use an electrode material that will corrode, even if the corrosion products are not toxic, because then the "battery" life will still be limited by the life of the electrode. This limits the possible electrode materials even further.

Talaat [7] has described a method for generating electricity that seems to circumvent many of these problems. His procedure takes advantage of the fact that the concentrations of oxygen in the right ventricle and in the aorta differ by a factor of approximately 2. Thus, by putting identical electrodes (made of platinum black) in these two sites, he is able to make a "concentration cell" and generate on the order of 100 μW of electricity, which is more than enough to operate a pacemaker. At the present time the principal drawback to this procedure seems to be the difficulty in inserting the electrodes into the proper places and making them stay fixed.

The thermodynamic approach to power generation would best be exemplified by thermocouples, which almost seems an obvious method. The problem here is the lack of a cold junction in the body. The body has an efficient temperature regulating system, which holds all points in the body to a narrow temperature range. The number of thermocouples required to generate sufficient electricity for a pacemaker would require an exorbitant amount of space. The outside of the body cannot be used for a cold junction because the external temperature is of the same order of magnitude as the body temperature and can even exceed it on a hot day, thus reversing the roles of the hot and cold junctions. At any rate, the external temperature is too variable to be relied on for this purpose.

A promising method of attacking this problem is to create an artificial hot junction for thermocouples with radioisotopes. The proposed isotope-powered cardiac pacemaker will use plutonium 238 at approximately 300°F to serve as the hot junction of a thermocouple system, with the body itself serving as the cold junction. Plutonium 238, with a half-life of almost 90 years, was selected because its principal emission is alpha rays, which can be stopped by the metal can of the container. Any material that had appreciable amounts of other emissions (such as gamma radiation) would require lead shielding to be acceptable in the body, and the amount of shielding required would produce a device with a prohibitive weight and volume. The hot junction temperature to be used for this device is an indication of the futility of trying to use thermocouples with normal differences in body temperatures at different points in the body, since the normal differences (of 2 or 3 degrees) are much smaller than the 200°F difference with the isotope-powered pacemaker. Furthermore, even the isotope-powered pacemaker does not produce a great surplus of power. The use of an artificial hot junction permits more efficient placement of thermocouples than would be possible if the temperature differences in the body alone were to be used. The use of an alpha emitter almost completely removes any radiation danger. Actually, some extra radiation could be permitted, since most pacemaker patients are older than 50 years.

2. ARTIFICIAL HEARTS

The power supply problem for the artificial heart is complicated because the requirement for these devices is on the order of 30 watts, instead of the milliwatts required for pacemakers. Thus it appears that biological sources of energy will not be feasible, because the required energy is not available inside the body. Research is currently concentrated on methods of bringing power from an external source into the body, rather than using an implanted battery or generating energy in the body. At present there is no battery that could supply 30 watts and would last for any appreciable length of time.

Many of the artificial hearts discussed previously require compressed air for their power source. With the present state of air compressors the source of air itself would have to be external, and the air would have to be introduced into the body through an opening in the skin. This does not seem feasible for long-term clinical use. Aside from the inconvenience of a permanent external attachment, openings in the skin invariably lead to infection.

Connectors for bringing power through the skin have been developed that tend to avoid infection if no stress is placed on them. These are basically plastic plugs with some material, such as Dacron mesh, placed around them so that the skin tends to grow into the plug. The holes themselves are often labyrinthine, to minimize the chance of foreign material passing through them. The holes are generally filled with silicone rubber after the necessary connections have been made. However, the connection to the skin is somewhat tenuous at best, and, as just mentioned, sudden stress or pulling will tend to create an opening.

The technique that seems most promising at this time is to transmit power through the skin by means of electromagnetic induction. The earliest developer of this technique was Schuder [8, 9], who used a frequency of 465 kHz and two "pancake" coils—one on the outside, and one on the inside, of the body. With this configuration he managed to transmit 38 watts of power with an efficiency of 95 percent. By markedly decreasing the efficiency he has developed a method by which the external coil does not have to be attached to the body. A device of this type has been tested experimentally in dogs [7]. It is shown schematically in Figure 12.5. Three orthogonal coils, 2 meters on an edge, surround the region to which the animal is restricted, and are excited at slightly different frequencies: 422, 425, and 428 kHz. As the animal moves around the relative position and orientation of its implanted coil with respect to the external coil set changes, but at any given time one or more of the external coils are supplying energy to the coil within the dog. The energy supplied varies with position and orientation, and the figures indicated in the drawing are approximate values for the most unfavorable position of the receiving coil when it is constrained to remain within the 1-m^3 region within the external coil set. The internal coil has a diameter of 9 cm. Such a device would be most useful for nonambulatory patients, who must remain within a limited physical area.

An approach that uses electromagnetic induction but at lower frequencies has been followed by Myers and Reed [10]. The device is illustrated in Figure 12.6. Two ferrite cup cores act as the primary and secondary of a transformer, with one core (and coil) implanted and the other strapped on ex-

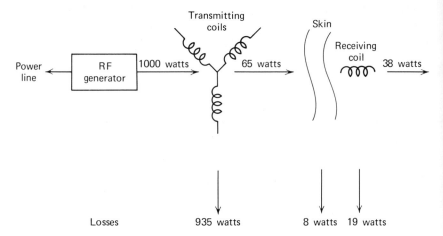

Figure 12.5 Method of coupling to implanted coils using radio-frequency energy at 455 kHz.

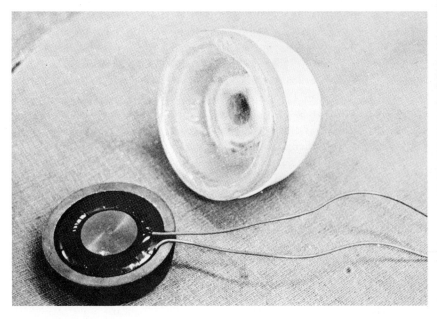

Figure 12.6 Coil used for coupling energy to implanted artificial heart using electromagnetic induction at 13 kHz.

ternally. The cores are 6 cm in diameter and weigh 8 oz. The frequency is 13 kHz. The primary and secondary are tuned by means of capacitors, and the coupling is adjusted so that at normal separation the two coils are slightly overcoupled. Thus, if misalignment should occur because of slipping of the strap or any other reason, the coupling coefficient will approach the critical value. Since both power transfer and efficiency have a small variation with coupling coefficient in this range, a considerable amount of misalignment is possible without seriously degrading power transfer. The power transfer and efficiency remained constant to within ±10 percent for a variation in air-gap spacing of from 8 to 17 mm, and a lateral motion of the cores of ±1 cm. The overall efficiency is 91 percent.

Since no batteries are presently available that will provide 30 watts for any reasonable length of time, the source of power can only be commercial electrical outlets. However, an artificial heart would not be a desirable prosthetic if the patient always had to be connected to a wall outlet, so research is being conducted to determine methods of temporarily storing energy in the body. One obvious method is to use a storage battery, which can be periodically charged from a wall outlet. The recharging period might be a few hours, which is not too desirable but still permits the patients a certain amount of freedom.

Another method being investigated is to convert electrical energy to heat, which is stored in a heat sink; this can be made fairly efficient. A heat engine would then convert the heat into a form suitable for the artificial heart. Isotope energy sources are also being explored for these applications, but here the radiation becomes a problem because of the thousandfold difference in the energy requirements of a heart as compared to a pacemaker. The advanced age of most patients who might require an artificial heart may prove to be important, because such patients do not have a very great life expectancy anyway and are usually well past the child-bearing age. If it is a choice between no chance of survival without the prosthetic, and a decreased life expectancy with it because of the radiation, then it may be reasonable to implant a device with more radiation than would be used with a younger person.

3.   DETECTION OF IMPENDING PACEMAKER FAILURE

The relatively short life of batteries in present use has influenced the design of pacemakers. In most pulse circuits it is considered desirable to have the rate independent of battery voltage, and most early pacemakers were designed with this in mind. However, it soon became apparent that if the rate were made to vary with battery voltage, a simple check could be made of the remaining life of the pacemaker, since the patient himself can easily take his pulse. Thus most pacemakers are now being designed so that the rate will vary with battery voltage.

It has also been found that if the electrocardiogram is measured with a wide-band oscilloscope, the pacemaker pulse appears in its true shape (undistorted by polarization) and undergoes an attenuation that depends only on the relative geometry of the pacemaker electrodes and the pickup electrodes of the electrocardiograph. Thus, if the electrocardiogram is periodically measured in this way from the time of implantation, the pulse amplitude, which is directly related to the battery voltage, can be followed; the pacemaker can be replaced after the pulse amplitude has dropped enough to indicate that the batteries may be failing. Since many pacemakers have a pulse shape that depends on the load resistance, such a method can also often detect cases where a pacemaker electrode has either become partially dislodged or is not making good contact. (If no contact is made, then the pacemaker will not pace, and the pacemaker or the electrodes must be replaced.) Such periodic pacemaker checkups are quite important, permitting elective replacement of a defective pacemaker in 50 to 75 percent of cases.

REFERENCES

[1] Parsonnet, V., G. Myers, I. R. Zucker, H. Lotman, and M. M. Asa, "A Cardiac Pacemaker Using Biologic Energy Sources," *Trans. ASAIO,* 9:174 (1963).

[2] Myers, G. H., V. Parsonnet, I. R. Zucker, and H. Lotman, "Biologically Energized Cardiac Pacemaker," *Am. J. Med. Elec.,* 3:233 (1964).

[3] Enger, C., and J. Kennedy, "An Improved Bioelectric Generator," *Trans. ASAIO,* 10:373 (1964).

[4] Strohl, C., R. Scott, W. Frezel, and S. Wolfson, "Studies of Bioelectric Power Sources for Cardiac Pacemakers," ibid., 12:318 (1966).

[5] Reynolds, W. L., "Utilization of Bioelectricity as a Power Supply for Electronic Devices," *Aerospace Med.,* 35:115 (1964).

[6] Roy, O. Z., and R. W. Wehnert, "Keeping the Heart Alive with a Biological Battery," *Electronics,* 39:105 (1966).

[7] Talaat, M., J. Kraft, R. Cowley, and A. Khazei, in "Biological Electrical Power," extraction from "Blood to Power Cardiac Pacemakers," *IEEE Trans. on Bio. Med. Eng.,* BME-14:263 (1967).

[8] Schuder, J. C., H. G. Stephenson, and J. F. Townsend, "High-Level Electromagnetic Energy Transfer Through a Closed Chest Wall."

[9] Schuder, J. C., and H. G. Stephenson, Jr., "Energy Transport with the Closed Chest from a Set of Very Large Mutually Orthogonal Coils," *Comm. and Elec.* 64:527 (1963).

[10] Myers, G. H., G. G. Reed, A. Thumim, S. Fascher, and L. Cortes, "A Transcutaneous Power Transformer," *Trans. Am. Soc. Art. Int. Organs,* XIV:210 (1968).

APPENDIX A

Electronic Circuit Elements

This appendix outlines briefly, for those unfamiliar with them, the nature and function of the principal electronic circuit elements currently in use in medical instruments. It is expected that the material will be completely familiar to all readers with an engineering background, who can omit reading it.

Circuit elements are usually classified either as active or passive. An active device, such as the transistor or vacuum tube, modulates a large power source and produces an output that depends on a low-power signal. Thus the active devices typically provide amplification of some sort. The passive devices, by contrast, have no external source of power applied to them and act merely to change the nature of the signal being applied.

The three common passive components are the resistor, the capacitor, and the inductor. These are defined in the following way:

The voltage across a resistor is proportional to the current through it. Thus, if V is the voltage across the resistor, I is the current through it in amperes, and R is the value of the resistance in ohms, then $V = IR$, which is familiar to most readers as Ohm's law.

The current through a capacitor is proportional to the rate of change of voltage across it. Thus, if I is the current through the capacitor in amperes, dV/dt is the rate of change of voltage across it in volts per second, and C is the value of the capacitance in farads, then $I = C \, dV/dt$.

The voltage across an inductor is proportional to the rate of change of current through it. If V is the voltage across an inductor in volts, dI/dt is the rate of change of current through the inductor in amperes per second, and L is the value of the inductance in henrys, then $V = L \, dI/dt$.

These relationships are illustrated graphically in Figure A.1. The symbols for all three components have been indicated, along with the standard conventions relating the sign of the voltage across the component to the direction of the current through it. For a resistor the current is shown increasing according to the formula $I = at$, so that the current has a constant rate of change. The voltage also has a constant rate of change, but its slope is proportional to the

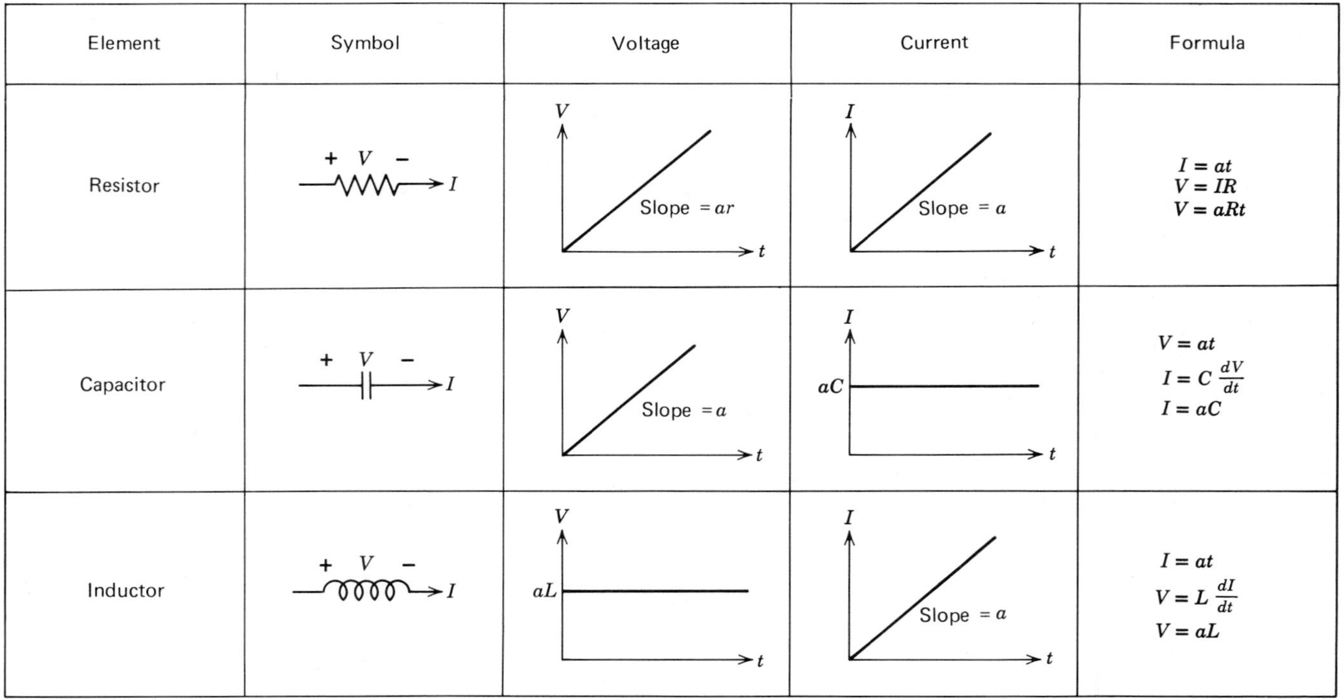

Element	Symbol	Voltage	Current	Formula
Resistor	+ V − ⟋⟍⟋⟍ → I	Slope = ar	Slope = a	$I = at$ $V = IR$ $V = aRt$
Capacitor	+ V − ⊣⊢ → I	Slope = a	aC	$V = at$ $I = C\dfrac{dV}{dt}$ $I = aC$
Inductor	+ V − ⦚⦚⦚ → I	aL	Slope = a	$I = at$ $V = L\dfrac{dI}{dt}$ $V = aL$

Figure A-1 Static and dynamic characteristics of ideal circuit elements.

value of the resistor. If the voltage across the capacitor has a constant rate of change equal to a (the slope of the line), then the current through the capacitor will be constant. The inductor presents exactly the dual relationship: the voltage across it is constant when the current has a constant rate of change.

These components, as they are defined here, are ideal components: no actual inductor follows these laws exactly; for example, an inductor is usually made by winding wire in a coil. Since the wire must always have some resistance, any actual inductor exhibits both resistance and inductance. Similarly, many resistors are made by winding wire into a coil, and thus have inductance. The usefulness of the concept of the ideal circuit element is that many actual components conform closely to these definitions, and those that do not can usually be represented as a combination of these elements (as in the case of the inductor and resistor just mentioned).

Actual sources of electricity are devices such as batteries or electrical generators. However, ideal sources may also be defined and are useful in analyzing circuits. The usual types of sources are the ideal voltage source and the ideal current source. By definition the ideal voltage source always has the same voltage across its terminals, whereas the ideal current source always has a constant output of current. That these ideal components are not physically realizable is immediately obvious, since any real source has no voltage output if it is short-circuited and no current output if it is open-circuited. Most physical sources can be represented by an ideal source and a resistor. Such a representation would consist either of a voltage source with a series resistor, or a current source with a parallel resistor. If an actual voltage source is very close to an ideal one, then the series resistor would be very small (ideally approaching zero); whereas in the case of the current source the parallel resistor would be very large, ideally approaching infinity. For this reason physical voltage sources are often called low-resistance (or low-impedance) sources, and physical current sources are called high-resistance (or high-impedance) sources. The question always arises in such cases: high (or low) with respect to what? In this case the source resistance would be high or low as compared to the load on the source. If the source resistance is about the same order of magnitude as the load, then it is not possible to consider the source as either a voltage source or a current source.

An important distinction between resistors on one hand, and capacitors and inductors on the other, is that resistors dissipate power, whereas capacitors and inductors store energy. Energy (measured in joules) is the capacity for doing work and has the same physical units as work. Power is the rate of change of energy. Thus, if a certain number of joules of energy are stored in a capacitor, then that number of joules can be used to perform useful work.

The power dissipated in a resistor (measured in watts, or joules per second) is given by $P_R = VI = V^2/R = I^2R$, where V and I are the voltage across and the current through the capacitor, respectively. The energy stored in a capacitor at any time is given by $U_c = \frac{1}{2}\,CV^2$, where C is the value of the capacitor in farads and V is the voltage across the capacitor. The energy stored in an inductor at any time is given by $U_L = \frac{1}{2}\,LI^2$, where L is the value of the inductance in henrys and I is the current through the inductor.

It is apparent from the preceding definitions that it is much easier to perform computations with resistive circuits than with those containing inductors and capacitors, since with resistive circuits we can use Ohm's law, whereas with inductors and capacitors we have complicated relationships involving rates of change. The concept of impedance is an attempt to improve this situation. Impedances may be used when the voltages and currents in an electrical network are all sinusoidal (direct current would be considered a special case of sinusoidal voltage with the frequency zero). Although this seems to be somewhat restrictive, by use of a Fourier series any periodic waveform can be represented as a sum of sinusoids, and then the impedances can be used separately for each harmonic in the series.

Figure A.2 shows what happens when a sinusoidal voltage source is applied to a network consisting of resistors, inductors, and capacitors. The voltage is given by $V = \sqrt{2}\,V_0 \sin 2\pi ft$. The current that results will be different in magnitude and will have its zero-crossings, or phase, different; it can be represented by $I = \sqrt{2}\,I_0 \sin (2\pi ft - \theta)$. (The reason for having

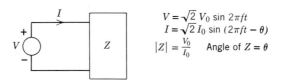

$$V = \sqrt{2}\,V_0 \sin 2\pi ft$$
$$I = \sqrt{2}\,I_0 \sin (2\pi ft - \theta)$$
$$|Z| = \frac{V_0}{I_0} \qquad \text{Angle of } Z = \theta$$

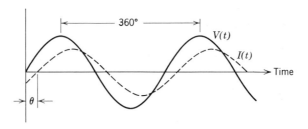

Figure A-2   Definition of generalized impedance for sinusoidal waves.

the factor $\sqrt{2}$ will be discussed later.) The impedance of the network, denoted by Z, allows us to compute the current given the voltage, or vice versa. Since there is both an amplitude change and a phase shift, the definition of Z must include two numbers. The magnitude of Z is equal to V_0/I_0, and what is called the angle of Z is given by θ. The angle theta can be put in degrees by considering one complete cycle to be 360 degrees and taking the ratio of θ to one full period. The relationship to be used for computing currents and voltages is then $V = IZ$.

1. The magnitude of V is given by the magnitude of I multiplied by the magnitude of Z.
2. The angle of V is given by the angle of I plus the angle of Z.

If the voltage is given and it is desired to compute the current, then $I = V/Z$ is used. The rules here are the following:

1. The magnitude of I equals the magnitude of V divided by the magnitude of Z.
2. The angle of I equals the angle of V minus the angle of Z.

Impedances may also be represented as complex numbers. In the case just discussed we could represent Z as $Z = A + jB$, where $j = \sqrt{-1}$, the magnitude of Z would equal $\sqrt{A^2 + B^2}$, and the angle of Z would equal $\tan^{-1}B/A$. The voltage and current would then also be complex numbers, where in all cases the magnitude of the complex number is the magnitude of the quantity concerned and the angle of the complex number is the angle of the quantity concerned.

It is conventional to use the factor $\sqrt{2}$ with sinusoidal magnitudes. The power supplied by a source of direct current is equal to VI, where V and I are the magnitudes of the voltage and current concerned. However, with a sinusoidal source, if V_p and I_p are the peak values of the sinusoid and the load is resistive, then the power is given by $\frac{1}{2} V_p I_p$. By including the $\sqrt{2}$ in the definitions we may say that even with a sinusoidal source the power is given by $V_0 I_0$ if the load is resistive. If the load is not resistive, then the average power dissipated is given by $V_0 I_0 \cos \theta$.

Up to this point only the passive circuit elements have been discussed. A basic description of the operation of the vacuum tube and transistor follows.

Figure A.3 shows a highly simplified version of the triode vacuum tube, where all of the elements have been shown in cross section and all have been put in a plane. Thus the cathode, grid, and anode would be flat pieces of metal extending into the paper. In actual construction practice these elements are usually concentric cylinders. The operation of the tube is as follows:

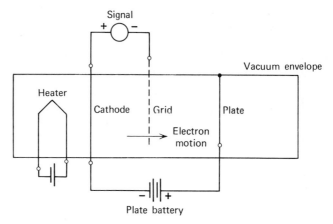

Figure A-3   Schematic representation of vacuum tubes.

1. An external battery powers a heating element, which raises the temperature of the cathode.

2. The elevated temperature of the cathode causes electrons to "boil off" the surface.

3. These electrons are attracted to the anode by the positive potential of the anode battery.

If a negative potential is applied to the grid, the number of electrons reaching the plate is diminished because the negative grid repels some electrons; thus the current in the anode circuit will vary in accordance with the grid voltage. Very little current is drawn by the grid circuit because the grid is not heated, and thus very few free electrons can become detached. Note, however, that if the grid becomes positive with respect to the cathode, it starts attracting the electrons passing through the tube, and substantial current is drawn through the grid circuit. If, however, the grid remains negative with respect to the cathode, there is very little grid current; thus very little power is drawn from the signal while there is substantial power in the output. Thus considerable power amplification results. If the grid voltage is made sufficiently negative, then almost all of the electrons leaving the cathode can be suppressed, and the tube is cut off. This mode of operation in which the tube is used basically as a switch is employed in counters and digital devices, where only two possible states are considered: conducting or not conducting. The vacuum tube without a grid can act as a diode. It is apparent that if the polarity of the battery on the anode is reversed, no current will flow because all of the electrons excited from the cathode will be repelled. Thus, current can only flow in one direction.

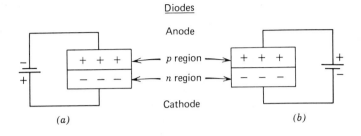

Diodes

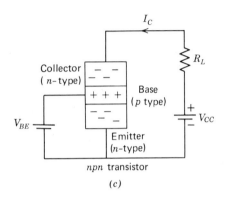

Figure A-4   Schematic representation of diodes and npn transistors: (*a*) reverse bias; (*b*) forward bias.

A transistor relies on the fact that there are free charge carriers in certain semiconductor materials. These charge carriers are analogous to the electrons in a vacuum tube, except that it is possible to have both positive and negative charge carriers, whereas in a vacuum tube only negative charge carriers (electrons) can be realized. If a semiconductor material has negative charge carriers, it is called *n*-type. If it has positive charge carriers, it is called *p*-type.

Figures A.4*a* and *b* show how a semiconductor diode works, in extremely oversimplified form. A *p* region and an *n* region are formed in a piece of semiconducting material. If the battery is connected as shown in Figure A.4*a* the positive carriers flow to the negative terminal of the battery and the negative charges flow to the positive terminal, with the result that no net current flows. This is called reverse bias. If the battery is reversed, then the positive and negative carriers are forced toward each other to the junction, where they combine with each other, permitting more carriers to flow in. Thus, a large current flows.

An *npn* transistor, shown in Figure A.4*c* has two junctions. Carriers are liberated in the emitter, diffuse across the *p*-type base, and then flow through the collector. Two junctions are present at the interfaces in the base. By changing the base voltage, the bias conditions at the junctions can be changed, altering the number of carriers that cross to the collector. Note that the base-emitter junction is forward biased, whereas the base-collector junction is reverse biased. Thus many carriers are attracted into the base region, but the reverse-biased collector junction tends to repel some of them. Thus the action is similar to that of a vacuum tube, with the emitter corresponding to the cathode, the base corresponding to the grid, and the collector corresponding to the anode. In the case of a transistor, however, current is usually drawn

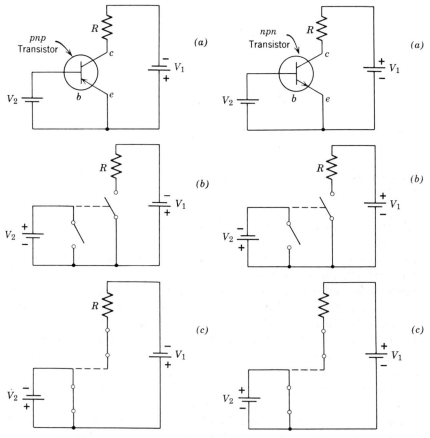

Figure A-5 Schematic representation of operation of an npn switching transistor: (*a*) basic circuit; (*b*) V_2 negative; (*c*) V_2 positive.

Figure A-6 Operation of *pnp* switching transistor: (*a*) basic circuit; (*b*) V_2 positive; (*c*) V_2 negative.

by the base circuit, so some power must be supplied at the input. If V_{BE}, the base-emitter voltage, is reversed in polarity, then the base-emitter junction is back biased, and very little current flows. This corresponds to cutoff in a vacuum tube, and is also used in digital devices and electronic switches. In a *pnp* transistor the collector and emitter are *p*-type, and the base is *n*-type. The methods of operation are exactly the same, but the polarities of all of the batteries must be reversed to properly bias the junctions. This feature has some advantages in certain applications.

Figures A.5 and A.6 show how *npn* and *pnp* transistors are used as switches. Part *a* of each figure shows the conventional symbol for each type of transistor, with the proper polarities of all batteries shown for amplifier operation. In part *b* the polarity of the emitter-base voltage is reversed, thus acting to open the switch, indicated schematically by open mechanical switches. Reversing the polarity to make it like that in part *c*, and making the base-emitter voltage sufficiently large has the effect of closing the switch, as is indicated in the figure. This principle is widely used in all pacemakers and also in digital devices.

The last major circuit component to be considered is the transformer, which changes voltages and currents. It is also a passive element. The "ideal" transformer, which can often be approximated in practice, is illustrated in Figure A.7. The symbol for it is two adjacent coils of wire with a dot at one end of each coil. A voltage v_1 is applied to the "primary" side; as a result, a voltage v_2 appears at the "secondary" side, where a resistive load has been indicated. The current flowing into the primary transformer is i_1, and the current emerging from the secondary side is i_2. If the turns ratio, or the ratio of the number of turns in the secondary winding to that in the primary winding, is n, then

$$v_2 = nv_1; \quad i_2 = i_1/n.$$

Note that the powers at the input and output, v_1i_1 and v_2i_2, are equal. As much power emerges from an ideal transformer as enters it.

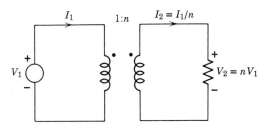

Figure A-7 Operation of ideal transformer.

If a transformer has an iron core (which makes it more efficient at low frequencies) it is customary to draw vertical lines between the coils. Because the transformer is basically two coils of wire in proximity it is possible to reverse the polarity of the secondary. The dots are used to indicate the actual connection. The convention is that current flows into a dot on the primary side and flows out of a dot on the secondary side. The dots then correspond to the positive terminals of both primary and secondary.

APPENDIX B

Additional Proofs

The purpose of this appendix is to justify the substitution in (2) of Chapter Five the insertion of the second derivative of the potential in the medium for the second derivative of the potential in the core of the cell. The differential equation governing the potential difference across the cell membrane if the cell is lying along a radial line extending from the electrode is

$$V = \lambda^2 \frac{d^2v}{dr^2} - v, \qquad (A\text{--}1)$$

where V is the voltage in the intracellular medium at r, and v is the potential inside the membrane. Both V and v are functions of r. We wish to show that

$$\frac{d^2V}{dr^2} \simeq \frac{d^2v}{dr^2} \qquad (A\text{--}2)$$

for the case $r >> \lambda$. Since r is about 2 mm and the electrode radii usually used for most pacemakers are much larger, this limitation has no practical significance. The proof here will be carried out for a cylindrical electrode. The proof for the spherical electrode follows the same lines.

Consider the tissue to be a uniform medium with conductivity σ. Then the current density $\mathbf{j}$ is given by

$$\mathbf{j} = \frac{-I}{2\pi r l}\, \mathbf{u}_r, \qquad (A\text{--}3)$$

where I is the total current through the electrode, l is its length, and $\mathbf{u}_r$ is the unit vector in the r direction. The electric field $\mathbf{E}$ is then

$$\mathbf{E} = -\sigma \mathbf{J} = \frac{-\sigma I}{2\pi l}\, \frac{\mathbf{u}_r}{r}. \qquad (A\text{--}4)$$

Let

$$C = \frac{\sigma I}{2\pi l};$$

then

$$\mathbf{E} = -C\, \frac{\mathbf{u}_r}{r}. \qquad (A\text{--}5)$$

Using the well-known fact that the electric field is the gradient of the potential and that this problem has cylindrical symmetry, it is then apparent that the potential in the medium is given by

$$V = C \ln r. \tag{A-6}$$

Using this solution with (A–1), the homogeneous solution may easily be shown to be

$$v_h = C_1 e^{r/\lambda} + C_2 e^{-r/\lambda}. \tag{A-7}$$

From general boundary conditions, and considering the fact that the heart is much bigger than the electrode, it is apparent that C_1 must be zero. It may be seen then that the homogeneous solution becomes very small if the radius r is much greater than the characteristic length λ.

The particular solution for v, the potential in the core of the cell, may be found in a straightforward manner by the method of variation of parameters. The result is shown in the next equation.

$$v_p = C \ln r - \frac{C}{2} \left(e^{r/\lambda} \int \frac{e^{-r/\lambda}}{r} \, dr + e^{-r/\lambda} \int \frac{e^{r/\lambda}}{r} \, dr \right). \tag{A-8}$$

Note that the first term in the expression for the particular solution is equal to the homogeneous solution. Thus, it is only necessary to show that the second part of this expression (the part in parentheses) has a second derivative with respect to r which vanishes for r much greater than λ. Note that the integrals in this expression cannot be evaluated in closed form. Although series solutions would be possible, it seems preferable to use the approximation previously indicated if it is at all valid, since then the total answer can be put in a relatively simple form.

The second derivative may easily be shown to be

$$\frac{d^2 v_p}{dr^2} = \frac{d^2 V}{dr^2} + \left[\int \frac{e^{-r/\lambda}}{r/\lambda} \, d(r/\lambda) \right] \frac{e^{r/\lambda}}{\lambda^2} + \left[\int \frac{e^{r/\lambda}}{r/\lambda} \, d(r/\lambda) \right] \frac{e^{-r/\lambda}}{\lambda^2}. \tag{A-9}$$

Since r is greater than λ, the well-known inequality

$$\int \frac{e^{r/\lambda}}{r/\lambda} \, d(r/\lambda) < \int e^{r/\lambda} \, d(r/\lambda) \tag{A-10}$$

will hold. If the substitution of (A–10) is made in (A–9), the integrals may be directly evaluated. If this is done, the result will be that

$$\frac{d^2 v_p}{dr^2} = \frac{d^2 V}{dr^2}.$$

Of course, this direct equality is due to the approximations made and the fact that an exact cancellation occurs. Since the actual products are always smaller than this and they decrease for increasing radius, it may be seen that the bracketed terms will decrease as the radius increases; and, since all these terms are functions of r/λ, then this will be true for $r > \lambda$.

Equivalent results can be shown by making a series expansion of the integrands, integrating them term by term, and multiplying by the series of expansions of the terms outside the brackets. In this case the terms will decrease as the radius increases, as has been indicated. The algebra is much more complex; however, the net result is equivalent to the one shown here by simpler means.

The Electrocardiogram

The electrical activity of the heart, as detected on an electrocardiogram, through surface skin electrodes, is seen in Figure C.1. The *P* wave, which represents depolarization of the atria, is followed after a short delay by the *QRS* complex, or depolarization of the ventricles. Essentially, the *P* wave is synonymous with atrial and the *QRS* complex, with ventricular contraction (see Chapter Nine). Depolarization of the ventricle is represented by the *T* wave. (The *T* wave of the atrium is "lost" in the *QRS* complex but can be seen if desired on intracardiac leads.)

In complete heart block, in which the electrical excitation wave of the atria does not reach the ventricles, the ventricles beat at their own intrinsic and relatively slow rate. Note in Figure C.1 the dissociation between the *P* wave and the *QRS* complexes.

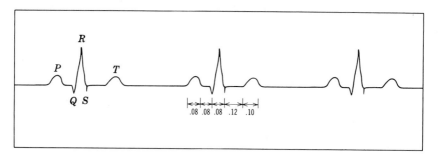

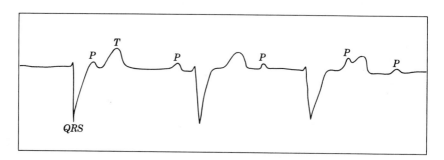

Figure C.1   The normal electrocardiogram, diagrammatic (upper trace), compared with that of complete heart block for which pacemakers are used: (*a*) Normal electrocardiogram (times in seconds); (*b*) electrocardiogram with heart block.

Index